Second Edition

Essentials of
Blood Banking and
Transfusion Medicine

*For Undergraduate and Postgraduate Students of
Medical Sciences, AYUSH, Laboratory Medicine and
Allied Health Sciences, and Clinicians in Practice*

Second Edition

Essentials of
Blood Banking and
Transfusion Medicine

*For Undergraduate and Postgraduate Students of
Medical Sciences, AYUSH, Laboratory Medicine and
Allied Health Sciences, and Clinicians in Practice*

Ganga S Pilli MD, PhD, DTM

Professor
Department of Pathology
JN Medical College
KLE Academy of Higher Education and Research
Belgaum, Karnataka

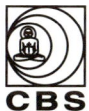

CBS

CBS Publishers & Distributors Pvt Ltd

New Delhi • Bengaluru • Chennai • Kochi • Kolkata • Lucknow • Mumbai
Hyderabad • Jharkhand • Nagpur • Patna • Pune • Uttarakhand

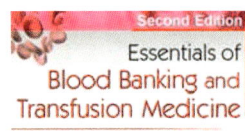

ISBN: 978-93-54660-31-3

Copyright © Author and Publisher

Second Edition: 2022
First Edition: 2012

Published by **Satish Kumar Jain** and produced by **Varun Jain** for

CBS Publishers & Distributors Pvt Ltd

4819/XI Prahlad Street, 24 Ansari Road, Daryaganj, New Delhi 110 002, India.
Ph: 011-23289259, 23266861, 23266867   Website: www.cbspd.com
Fax: 011-23243014   e-mail: delhi@cbspd.com;
          cbspubs@airtelmail.in.

Corporate Office: 204 FIE, Industrial Area, Patparganj, Delhi 110 092
Ph: 011-4934 4934   Fax: 011-4934 4935
          e-mail: publishing@cbspd.com; publicity@cbspd.com

Branches

- **Bengaluru:** Seema House 2975, 17th Cross, K.R. Road, Banasankari 2nd Stage, Bengaluru 560 070, Karnataka, India
  Ph: +91-80-26771678/79   Fax: +91-80-26771680   e-mail: bangalore@cbspd.com
- **Chennai:** 7, Subbaraya Street, Shenoy Nagar, Chennai 600 030, Tamil Nadu, India
  Ph: +91-44-26680620, 26681266   Fax: +91-44-42032115   e-mail: chennai@cbspd.com
- **Kochi:** 42/1325, 1326, Power House Road, Opp KSEB, Ernakulum, Kochi 682 018, Kerala, India
  Ph: +91-484-4059061-65,67   Fax: +91-484-4059065   e-mail: kochi@cbspd.com
- **Kolkata:** 147, Hind Ceramics Compound, 1st Floor, Nilgunj Road, Belghoria, Kolkata-700056, India
  Ph: +91-9096713055/7798394118, 9836841399   e-mail: kolkata@cbspd.com
- **Lucknow:** Basement, Khushnuma Complex, 7 Meerabai Marg (Behind Jawahar Bhawan), Lucknow-226001, UP, India
  Ph: +0522-4000032   e-mail: tiwari.lucknow@cbspd.com
- **Mumbai:** PWD Shed, Gala no 25/26, Ramchandra Bhatt Marg, Next to JJ Hospital Gate no. 2, Opp. Union Bank of India, Noorbaug, Mumbai-400009, Maharashtra, India
  Ph: +91-22-66661880/89   e-mail: mumbai@cbspd.com

Representatives

| • Hyderabad | 0-9885175004 | • Jharkhand | 0-9811541605 | • Nagpur | 0-9421945513 |
| • Patna | 0-9334159340 | • Pune | 0-9623451994 | • Uttarakhand | 0-9716462459 |

Printed at Nutech Print Services, Faridabad, Haryana, India

to

---

my parents and family members
and
my dear students who are my inspirers

Foreword

It gives me immense pleasure to write the Foreword to this book *Essentials of Blood Banking and Transfusion Medicine*. There are several elaborate as well as short textbooks on blood banking and blood transfusion, both Indian and foreign, but many of them do not have required up-to-date information. This book has been planned to give details of blood donation, techniques in blood banking, blood transfusion reactions, component therapy, blood transfusion in clinical practice, use of quality control and many other topics with recent advances.

Today, blood transfusion medicine is one of the rapidly expanding fields of medicine. This book is not only useful for students and technologists, but also to the practising physicians and surgeons, more so for the medical professionals working in the blood banks. The main purpose of this book is to provide easy and quick access to the information and guidelines on blood transfusion to the clinicians and all those who work with blood transfusion.

The author has chosen this subject to contribute her efforts with experience in diagnostic services in blood banking. This is the second edition of the book which speaks the popularity and demand of the book with updated information. I am sure it will be useful to all the students, both undergraduate and postgraduate, and clinicians, to achieve the goal of transfusion service to provide safe blood and blood components.

I congratulate the author for the pains she has taken to bring out the second edition of the book and wish her a great success.

VD Patil
Ex-Registrar
KLE University, Belagavi

Preface to the Second Edition

The book *Essentials of Blood Banking and Transfusion Medicine* now has seen the second edition with the help of CBS Publishers and Distributors. I am grateful to publishers for making this book to reach all my students not only locally but also nationally and internationally.

Though in brief, manuscript is prepared keeping in mind the necessary material both the theory and practical aspects required for the postgraduate students of pathology, clinical postgraduate students, clinicians, MBBS students, other medical students of AYUSH, Diploma and BSc (Laboratory Technology) students and nursing staff who work with blood. For the second edition of the book, four new chapters have been added and other chapters are updated.

I am grateful to Dr Shweta Nanjannavar and Dr Sangeeta Pathak for contributing following chapters to this book.

1. Chapter 20: "Motivation, recruitment and retention of blood donors" by Dr Shweta B Nanjannavar

2. Chapter 23: "Convalescent plasma and SARS-CoV-2 (COVID-19) antibodies" by Dr Sangeeta Pathak

I acknowledge all those who are directly or indirectly involved in preparation of the material for this book, especially my postgraduate and laboratory technology students.

I have made effort to give, at a glance, the necessary knowledge on blood banking and transfusion medicine which may be difficult for our readers to go through the voluminous books in transfusion medicine.

I am grateful to Dr Kavita GU, Professor of Pathology and Blood Bank In-charge at SS Institute of Medical Sciences, Davangere, for going through the manuscript of the second edition.

I appreciate the efforts and dedication of Mr SV Virgi for his valuable technical suggestions with his rich experience at blood bank.

I am thankful to Dr (Mrs) AV Dhaded, retired Professor of Pathology, Belgaum Institute of Medical Sciences, and former Professor and Head, Department of Pathology, for the critical appraisal of the book during infantile phase.

I am grateful to my children (Vijay and Veena), their spouses, and my husband Dr SC Pilli for their inspiration in preparation of the manuscript.

I am thankful to Dr Uday V Kokatnur for helping me in drawing the schematic and line diagrams.

More than all this, I thank my parents from whom I learnt the art of writing, especially my father who at the age of 84 is still an active writer in chosen field of his subject, and my mother supporting him in his endeavors.

Finally, I bow to all my superiors and Almighty.

Ganga S Pilli

Preface to the First Edition

This is my second book. I started writing material for this book two years back. I am grateful to all those who are directly or indirectly involved in preparation of the material for this book especially my postgraduate and laboratory technology students.

Though in brief, I have done this manuscript keeping in mind the necessary material both the theory and practical aspects required for the postgraduate students of pathology, clinical postgraduate students who utilize blood, clinicians, MBBS students, other medical students of Alternative System of Medicine, Diploma and B.Sc. (Laboratory Technology) students and nursing staff who work with blood.

I have made this effort to give, at a glance, the principles and practice of blood banking which may be difficult for our readers to go through the voluminous books in transfusion medicine.

I am grateful to Dr Sangeeta Pathak, Sr. Consultant and Head of Transfusion Medicine at Max Healthcare, New Delhi, for going through the material and giving the critical appraisal for the book.

I appreciate the efforts and dedication of Mr. SV Virgi, for his valuable technical suggestions with his rich experience at blood bank.

I am thankful to Dr. (Mrs.) AV Dhaded, Presently Professor, Department of Pathology, Belgaum Institute of Medical Sciences, for going through the material and giving the critical appraisal for the book.

I am grateful to our beloved registrar of KLE University, Dr VD Patil, Dr MV Jali, Medical Director and CE and Dr AS Godhi, Principal, JN Medical College, for giving me an opportunity and encouraging me to make this difficult task, a successful venture.

I fail in my duty if I do not express my gratitude to my children (Vijay and Veena) and husband Dr SC Pilli who tolerated me, when I was busy spending most of my time in preparation of the material at home or away at workplace and library.

More than all this, I thank my parents from whom I learnt the art of writing, especially my father who at the age of 75 is still an active writer in his chosen field of subject, and my mother supporting him in his endeavors.

Finally, I acknowledge the support from Chancellor Dr Prabhakar Kore, Vice-Chancellor Dr CK Kokate, *Ex*-Registrar Dr PF Kotur and bow to Almighty for his blessings.

Ganga S Pilli

Contents

Foreword by VD Patil   *vii*

Preface to the Second Edition   *ix*

Preface to the First Edition   *xi*

1. Safe Use of Blood   1

2. Blood Donation   15

3. Donor Health Screening, Donor Suitability Evaluation, Phlebotomy, Post-Donation Care and Adverse Donor Reactions   30

4. ABO Blood Group Systems   38

5. Subgroups of ABO System and Bombay Phenotype   55

6. Rh Typing and Weaker Variants of Rh System   58

7. Preparation and Standardization of Anti-Human Globulin (AHG) Reagent   63

8. Coombs' Test   66

9. Crossmatching   73

10. Transfusion Reactions   78

11. Transfusion Transmitted Diseases (TTDs)   95

12. Preservation of Blood, Principles and its Applications in Blood Banking   104

13. Blood and Blood Components   113

14. Blood Transfusion in Clinical Practice   124

15. Autologous Blood Transfusion   148

16. Blood Substitutes   152

17. HLA Antigens and other Platelet and Leucocyte Antigens and their Role in Blood Transfusion   156

18. Errors and Discrepancies in ABO Typing   162

19. Blood Bank Organization and its Management   171

20. Motivation, Recruitment and Retention of   182
     Blood Donors

21. Recent Advances in Blood Banking   188

22. Quality Improvement and Quality Control in   193
     Blood Transfusion Services

23. Convalescent Plasma and SARS-CoV-2   211
     (COVID-19) Antibodies

References   *217*

Index   *221*

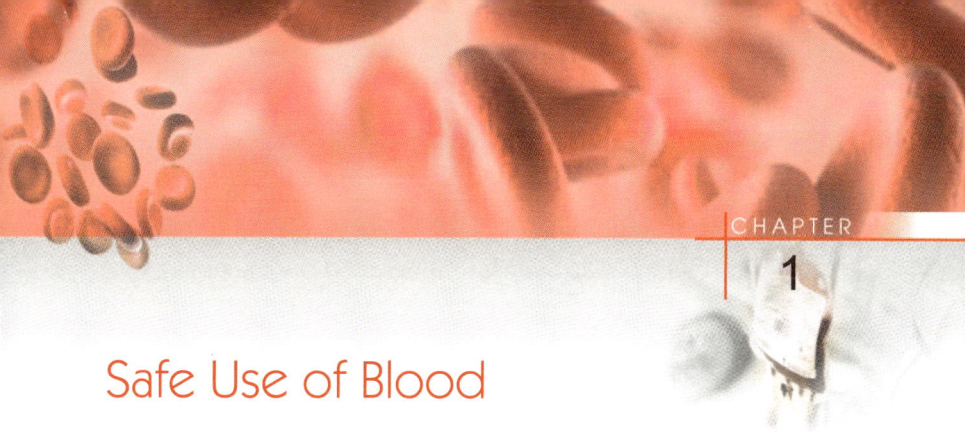

Safe Use of Blood

Before transfusing check the compatibility report, the label attached to the blood bag for the following:
- IP number
- Name of the patient including middle name and surname.
- The name and IP number should tally.
- Blood group.
- Donor registration number.
- Date of collection and date of expiry.

At the bedside confirm the patient's identity which should be checked from:
- The records of the patient.
- The patient himself verbally.
- In unconscious patients identify the patient from wrist band.

Following are the most important points:
1. Do not infuse any other medication along with blood.
2. A doctor should supervise the event.
3. When transfusing blood, watch the patient for first 15 minutes for vitals. Then watch every 30 minutes till transfusion is completed.
4. Rate of transfusion for whole blood/PRBCs should be 1 mL/minute and transfusion should be completed within 4 hours.
5. Avoid transfusion from family members in view of graft versus host disease (GVHD).

Blood transfusion is not without risks. Hence overweigh the benefits for the patient.

The reason for this is:
- Blood cannot be manufactured. It has to come only from **donors**.
- The red cells have antigens on their surface.
- In routine practice, it is necessary to determine the compatibility of certain red cell antigens between the donor and the recipient.
- Blood can be a source of blood transmitted infectious diseases.

There are many blood group systems. Amongst these, the two most important blood groups in blood transfusion are:
- ABO System
- Rh System

ABO and Rh compatible blood is mandatory requirement. Testing for rare blood groups can be sometimes encountered. **Do not transfuse unless clear indication is present. Some of the indications of blood transfusion are given below.**
- Chronic anaemias with Hb less than 6 gm/dL.
- Less than 7 gm/dL when patient is symptomatic and undergoing surgery.
- Less than 8 gm/dL with CVS problems.
- With 6–10 gm/dL only when severe bleeding or complications of inadequate hypoxia are expected.
- Blood loss of 30–40% of circulating blood volume (CBP).
- In anaemia/severe heart or pulmonary disease/when bleeding continues with blood loss of 15–30% of CBP.
- In obstetrics patients Hb less than 7 gm/dL, not amenable to timely therapies antenataly.
- In concealed haemorrhage with abruptio placenta, to replenish the concealed blood loss irrespective of symptoms.

Points to keep in mind for neonates:
- In neonates 10–20 mL/kg body weight blood can be given.
- Blood less than 7 days is preferred for neonatal transfusion.
- In neonates only antigen grouping is done.
- Blood to be given to neonate should be compatible with mother's serum.
- If mother's and baby's group are the same, use Rh negative blood of baby/mother's ABO group. If not the same, use 'O' Rh negative blood.

- In neonates, rate of transfusion should be 10–20 mL/kg to be given over 4 hours.

Points to keep in mind regarding transfusion
- One unit of whole blood will increase Hb by 1 gm/dL and PCV by 3%. 1 unit of packed red cells has 250 mg of iron.
- Iron that can be removed by the body is 1 mg/day.
- One unit of single donor platelets (SDP) will increase platelet count by 30,000–60000 platelets/cmm.
- One unit of random donor platelets (RDP) will increase the platelet count by 4,000–6000 platelets/cmm.
- Preserve the platelets at 22–24 degree C in agitator.
- Transfuse platelets, if platelet count is less than 10,000 cells/cmm. With antibodies to platelets, platelet transfusion may not be of use.
- Platelet increase is observed after 1 hour and again at 20–24 hours of platelet transfusion.
- Preserve the whole blood/PRBCs at 1–6 degree C.
- FFP once collected from the Blood Bank, can be preserved at 1–6 degree C and has to be used within 6 hours.

Observe for transfusion reactions (TR). These can be due to many reasons, e.g. alloantibodies, autoantibodies, complement activation, GVHD, etc. These can be classified as:

Acute transfusion reactions—immunological
- Febrile non-haemolytic transfusion reaction (FNHTR) allergic reactions
- Anaphylactic and anaphylactoid reactions
- Acute haemolytic transfusion reactions (AHTRs)
- Transfusion related acute lung injury (TRALI)

Acute transfusion reactions—non-immunological
- Bacterial contamination
- Transfusion—associated circulatory overload (TACO)
- Physical and chemical haemolysis
- Metabolic derangements

Delayed transfusion reactions—immunological
- Delayed haemolytic transfusion reaction (DHTR)

- Transfusion associated graft-versus-host disease (TA-GvHD)
- Post-transfusion purpura

Delayed transfusion reactions—non-immunological
- Iron overload
- Transfusion transmitted diseases

Immediate adverse effects of transfusion and their management

Category 1: Mild reactions			
Signs	*Symptoms*	*Possible cause*	*Immediate management*
Urticaria/ rash	Pruritis (itching)	Allergic	1. Stop transfusion 2. Assess patient 3. An antihistamine may be required 4. Transfusion may be restarted if no other signs/symptoms are present 5. If signs/symptoms worsen, treat as Category 2.

Category 2: Moderately severe reactions			
Signs	*Symptoms*	*Possible cause*	*Immediate management*
Flushing	Anxiety	Allergic (moderately-severe)	1. Stop transfusion and maintain IV line with normal saline
Urticaria	Pruritis	Febrile non-haemolytic transfusion reaction: Antibodies to white cells or platelets	2. Contact medical officer
Rigors	Palpitations		3. Patient may require antihistamine medication and/or paracetamol
Fever	Mild dyspnea	Antibodies to proteins including IgA	4. Further investigation and management according to clinical features
Restlessness	Headache	Possible contamination with pyrogens	
Tachycardia		and/or bacteria	If investigation required: Complete transfusion reaction form and send blood pack, form and samples to blood bank

(Contd.)

Category 3: Life-threatening reactions			
Signs	*Symptoms*	*Possible cause*	*Immediate management*
Rigors Fever Restlessness Hypotension	Anxiety Chest pain Pain at infusion site	1. Acute intra- vascular haemolysis (wrong blood)	1. Stop transfusion and maintain IV line with normal saline 2. Contact medical officer on duty
Tachycardia Dark Urine Unexplained bleeding (DIC)	Respiratory distress Loin/back pain Headache Dyspnea	2. Bacterial conta- mination and septic shock 3. Fluid overload 4. Anaphylaxis Transfusion related acute lung injury (TRALI)	3. Manage immediate needs: a. Fluid for hypotension b. Oxygen c. Adrenaline for ana-phylaxis d. Diuretic for fluid overload 4. Further management according to likely cause 5. Bedside clerical checks of all forms, labels and patient identification for correctness of the unit and the intended recipient are required. Reconfirm ABO, Rh and antibody screen and crossmatch tests. 6. Complete transfusion reaction form and the unit and all tubing should be returned to the blood bank, along with post-infusion blood and urine samples (DCT, urine hemoglobinuria, serum bilirubin, hemo-globinaemia, urea, creatinine, electrolytes, urine output, coagula-tion screen

(Contd.)

7. Additional samples sometimes required for (a) Blood cultures, (b) HLA or neutrophil antibodies, (c) Anti-IgA antibodies and (d) HLA typing
8. The reaction should be documented in the patient's chart. Once these initial measures have been implemented, the investigation of the reaction by the transfusion service can proceed

ACUTE HAEMOLYTIC REACTIONS

Causes

- The majority of haemolytic reactions are caused by transfusion of **ABO incompatible** blood, e.g. group A transfused to group B patient or vice versa.
- Antibodies in the patient's plasma will hemolyse the incompatible red cells.

Even a small volume of incompatible blood (5–10 mL) can cause severe reactions and large volumes increase the risk.

Symptoms: Chills, fever, pain (along IV line, back, chest), hypotension, dark urine, uncontrolled bleeding due to DIC.

The common cause of AHTR is transfusion of ABO incompatible blood and this can be due to:

- Errors in blood request form
- Taking wrong sample into prelabeled sample tube
- Incorrect labeling of the sample tube sent to the blood bank
- Inadequate checks of the blood against the identity of the patient while starting a transfusion
- In a conscious patient signs and symptoms appear within minutes of starting the transfusion; sometimes even less than 10 mL have been given.

- In an unconscious or anaesthetized patient, hypotension and uncontrolled bleeding (DIC) may be the only signs.
- Hence monitor the patient at the start of transfusion.

Prevention of Errors

1. Correctly label the blood samples and request forms.
2. Place the patient's blood sample in the sample tube.
3. Always check the blood against the identity of the patient at the bedside before transfusion.
4. Proper identification of the patient from sample collection through to blood administration, proper labeling of samples and products are essential. Prevention of non-immune haemolysis requires adherence to proper handling, storage and administration of blood products.

Management: Immediately stop transfusion. Notify hospital blood bank immediately (another patient may also have been given the wrong blood!). These patients usually require ICU support and therapy includes vigorous treatment of hypotension and maintenance of renal blood flow.

FEBRILE REACTIONS

This is the most common cause of TR.

Cause: Recipient antibodies reacting with white cell antigens or white cell fragments in the blood product or due to cytokines which accumulate in the blood product during storage. Fever occurs more commonly with platelet transfusion than red cell transfusion.

It is important to distinguish from fever due to the patient's underlying disease or infection (check pre-transfusion temperature). Fever may be the initial symptom in a more serious reaction such as bacterial contamination or haemolytic reaction and should be taken seriously.

Management
- If fever is present, give paracetamol.
- Follow the steps of 'immediate management' of an acute transfusion reaction. For isolated fever or chills in some

patients, the treating doctor may choose to restart the transfusion. If the fever is accompanied by significant changes in blood pressure or other signs and symptoms, the transfusion should be ceased and investigated.
- Check for HLA antibodies in patients having repeated febrile reactions.

Prevention: A proportion of patients who have febrile reactions will have similar reactions to subsequent transfusions. Many are prevented by pre-storage leucocyte filtration.

URTICARIAL (ALLERGIC) REACTIONS

Cause: Caused by **foreign plasma proteins**. On rare occasions, this is associated with laryngeal oedema and bronchospasm.

Management
- If urticaria occurs in isolation (without fever and other signs), slow the rate or temporarily stop transfusion.
- If symptoms are mild, administer **anti-histamine medication** before restarting the transfusion. If associated with other symptoms, cease the transfusion and proceed with investigation.

Investigation
In case of mild urticarial reactions with no other signs or symptoms, it is not necessary to submit blood specimens for investigation. It is also usually possible to restart the transfusion. Such a decision should be made after assessment by the treating doctor.

ANAPHYLACTIC/ANAPHYLACTOID REACTIONS

Anaphylactic and anaphylactoid reactions have signs of cardiovascular instability including hypotension, tachycardia, loss of consciousness, cardiac arrhythmia, shock and cardiac arrest. Sometimes respiratory involvement with dyspnea and stridor are prominent.

Cause: In some cases, patients with IgA deficiency, who have anti-IgA antibodies can have these reactions.

Management
- Immediately stop transfusion, supportive care including airway management may be required. Adrenaline may be indicated. Usually given as 1:1000 dilution, 0.01 mg/kg subcutaneously/IM or slow IV.
- **Investigate** for IgA levels and anti-IgA antibodies.

Prevention: Patients with anti-IgA antibodies require special blood products such as washed red blood cells and plasma products prepared from IgA deficient donors.

BACTERIAL CONTAMINATION

Cause: Bacteria may be introduced into the blood pack at the time of blood collection from sources such as donor skin, donor bacteraemia or equipment used during blood collection or processing. Bacteria may multiply during storage. Gram positive and Gram negative organisms have been implicated. **Platelets are more frequently implicated than red cells.**

Some contaminants, particularly **pseudomonas species grow at 2–6 degree C** and **staphylococci** grow at **20–24 degree C.**

Signs and symptoms appear rapidly after starting the infusion, but may be delayed for a few hours.

Symptoms: Common symptoms are very high fever, rigor, profound hypotension, nausea and/or diarrhoea. **A severe reaction may be characterized by sudden onset of high fever, rigors and hypotension.**

Management
- Immediately stop the transfusion and notify the hospital blood bank. After initial supportive care, blood cultures should be taken and high dose broad-spectrum anti-microbials need to be administered.
- Laboratory investigation will include culture of the blood pack.

Prevention
- Inspect blood products prior to transfusion. Some but not all bacterially contaminated products can be recognised (clots, clumps, or abnormal colour).

- Maintaining appropriate cold storage of red cells in a blood bank refrigerator is important.
- Transfusions should not proceed beyond the recommended infusion time (4 hours).

FLUID OVERLOAD

1. Fluid overload can result in heart failure and pulmonary oedema
2. May occur when:
   - Too much fluid is transfused.
   - The transfusion is too rapid.
   - Renal function is impaired.
3. Fluid overload is likely to occur in patients with
   - Chronic severe anaemia
   - Underlying cardiovascular disease

TRANSFUSION-RELATED ACUTE LUNG INJURY

Transfusion related acute lung injury (TRALI) is a clinical diagnosis of exclusion characterised by **acute respiratory distress and bilaterally symmetrical pulmonary oedema with hypoxaemia developing within 2 to 8 hours after a transfusion**. A chest X-ray shows interstitial or alveolar infiltrates when no cardiogenic or other cause of pulmonary oedema exists.

Cause: Pulmonary vascular effects are thought to occur secondary to cytokines in the transfused product or from interaction between patient's white cell antigens and donor antibodies (or vice versa).

Management
- **Symptomatic support for respiratory distress includes oxygen administration** and may require intubation and mechanical ventilation.
- Symptoms generally resolve over 24–48 hours.

HYPOTHERMIA

Cause: Rapid infusion of large volumes of stored blood contributes to hypothermia. Infants are particularly at risk during exchange or massive transfusion.

Prevention and management
- Appropriately maintained blood warmers should be used during massive or exchange transfusion.
- Additional measures include warming of other intravenous fluids and the use of devices to maintain patient body temperature.

HYPERKALEMIA

Cause: Stored red cells leak potassium proportionately throughout their storage life. Irradiation of red cells increases the rate of potassium leakage. Clinically significant hyperkalemia can occur during rapid, large volume transfusion of older red cell units in neonates and children.

Prevention: Red cells are irradiated just prior to issue especially in neonates and children. Blood less than 7 days old is generally used for transfusion in neonates (e.g. cardiac surgery, ECMO, exchange transfusion).

DELAYED HAEMOLYTIC TRANSFUSION REACTION (DHTR)[1]

DHTR commonly occurs after 24 hrs, may occur several days after administration of red cells usually from 2 to 14 days.

Cause: Patients may develop antibodies to red cell antigens. Antibodies can occur naturally, or may arise as a consequence of previous transfusion or pregnancy. A delayed haemolytic reaction occurs when a patient develops an antibody directed against an antigen on transfused red cells. The antibody may cause shortened red cell survival, with clinical features of fever, jaundice and lower than expected haemoglobin following transfusion.

Prevention: An antibody screen is performed as part of pre-transfusion testing. When an antibody is detected, it is identified and appropriate antigen negative blood is provided. Sometimes antibodies fall below detectable limits and may not be detected by pretransfusion testing.

TRANSFUSION ASSOCIATED GRAFT-VERSUS-HOST DISEASE (TA-GvHD)

Cause: TA-GvHD occurs from donor lymphocytes in a susceptible transfusion recipient. These donor lymphocytes proliferate and damage target organs especially bone marrow, skin, liver and gastrointestinal tract. The clinical syndrome comprises fever, skin rash, pancytopenia, abnormal liver function and diarrhoea and is fatal in over 80% of cases. **The usual onset is about 12 days of** post-transfusion period.

Also, can occur in immunocompetent recipients of blood from a biologically related (directed) or HLA identical donors. The disease is also reported in immunologically compromised patients.

Prevention: Gamma irradiation of cellular blood products (whole blood, red blood cells, platelets, granulocytes) for patients of risk group has to be given.

Risk groups

- Recipients of blood from biologically related (directed) or HLA matched donors.
- Patients with congenital immunodeficiency
- Patients receiving granulocyte transfusions
- Patients with Hodgkin's disease
- Allogeneic and autologous peripheral blood stem cell (PBSC) and bone marrow transplant recipients
- Patients with aplastic anaemia receiving immuno-suppression
- Patients treated with purine analogue drugs

Post-transfusion purpura: For details refer to transfusion reactions.

TRANSFUSION RELATED IMMUNE MODULATION (TRIM)

Allogenic blood transfusion may be associated with immuno-suppression, increased risk of infection and cancer recurrence.

Cause: Unknown, possibly mediated by donor white cells or plasma.

IRON ACCUMULATION

Cause: Iron accumulation is a predictable consequence of chronic RBC transfusion. Organ toxicity begins when reticulo-endothelial sites of iron storage become saturated. Liver and endocrine dysfunction creates significant morbidity and the most serious complication is cardiotoxicity which causes arrhythmias, and congestive heart failure. Patients receiving chronic transfusion should monitor their iron status monitored and managed by their physician.

Management and pevention: Iron chelation therapy is usually commenced early in the course of chronic transfusion therapy.

INFECTIOUS DISEASE TRANSMISSION

A variety of infectious agents may be transmitted by transfusion. Hence proper screening is essential.

ALLOIMMUNISATION

In this, the antibodies are formed to the antigens those are not present on the person's blood cells.

Red cell alloimmunization: Patients experiencing alloantibody formation are asymptomatic. The alloantibody is discovered at the time of pre-transfusion testing. Appropriate antigen negative blood should be supplied.

Prevention: Alloimmunisation to the D and K (Kell) antigens is prevented by the provision of Rh(D) negative and Kell negative blood for Rh(D) negative, Kell negative patients respectively. This is important for females with child-bearing potential as these antibodies can cause severe haemolytic disease of the newborn during pregnancy.

Risk groups: Patients with sickle cell disease or major haemo-globinopathy syndromes who are chronically transfused are at greatest risk of alloantibody formation. Prior to commencing transfusion, patients with these conditions should have extended red cell phenotyping performed. Blood matched for the patient's Rhesus and Kell antigens is usually supplied for transfusion

Platelet alloimmunization: When thrombocytopenic patients do not achieve the expected post-transfusion platelet count increment, they are said to be refractory. This usually occurs in patients receiving frequent platelet transfusions.

Causes: There are clinical and immunological causes of platelet refractoriness. Clinical causes include sepsis, DIC, bleeding, fever, some drugs, and enlarged spleen.

Immunological causes include the development of antibodies to human leucocyte antigens (HLA) or human platelet antigens (HPA).

Management: Immunological refractoriness can be managed by the provision of HLA or HPA matched platelets.

Prevention: Leucocyte reduction of blood and blood products to levels less than 10^6/unit reduces the likelihood of alloimmunisation. This can be achieved through the use of pre-storage or bedside leucocyte reduced blood products.

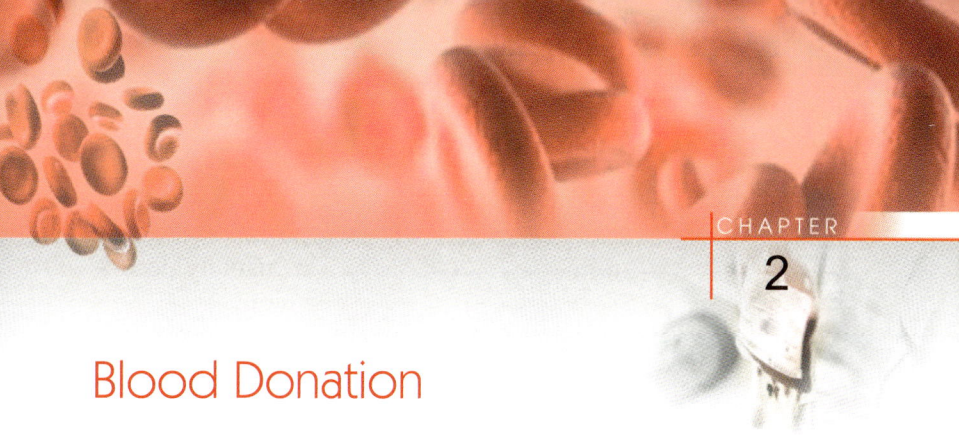

Blood Donation

IMPORTANCE OF BLOOD DONATION[2]

Following are some of the facts of blood transfusion:

- Every two seconds someone needs blood and it may be you.
- One out of ten patients in a hospital requires blood.
- According to WHO data in the South East Asian Region (SEAR) countries, the annual requirement is 15 million units, but collected is only 9.3 million units.[2] In India, every year our nation requires about 9–9.5 million units of blood, out of which only about 60% of blood is available.
- More than 1 million new patients are diagnosed with cancer each year. Many of them will need blood, sometimes daily, during their chemotherapy treatment.
- Blood cannot be manufactured. It has to come only from **generous donors**.
- Blood donation is the greatest donation. You are saving life, not one, but three to four lives.
- The average adult has 5 liters of blood in his body.
- **You are donating less than 500 mL of blood.**
- **About 8 mL per kg body weight blood can be given**.
- Donating blood is a safe process. A sterile needle is used to each donor and blood donation takes less than 10–12 minutes.
- **The donated red blood cells/whole blood is used within 35 days with CPDA1.**
- **Donated platelets are used within 5 days.**
- **Plasma and cryoprecipitate are stored in frozen state and can be used up to one year**.

AIMS OF BLOOD DONATION

The main aim of blood donation is to save the patients by blood transfusion in the following occasions:

- In emergency cases such as bleeding during accidents.
- Bleeding in disorders like haemophilia and other bleeding disorders.
- In cases of severe anaemias.
- In pregnant patients with bleeding before, during or after delivery.
- During major surgeries such as heart surgeries, etc.

Quantity of blood to be donated

The amount of blood to be drawn is determined by the following formula:

$$\text{Amount of blood to be drawn} = \frac{\text{Donor's weight in kg}}{50} \times 450$$

$$\text{Amount of blood to be drawn} = \frac{\text{Donor's weight in lbs}}{110} \times 450$$

You are donating 350 mL/450 mL (one unit) of blood and it is collected in appropriate anticoagulant (CPD-A1) to prevent coagulation. This represents 10–13% of blood volume which can be well sustained by our body.

For 100 mL of blood 14 mL of anticoagulant/preservative is added. The amount of anticoagulant needed for the specific volume to be drawn is calculated as follows:

Anticoagulant to be used

$$\text{Amount of anticoagulant} = \frac{\text{Amount of blood drawn}}{100} \times 14$$

Healthy bone marrow makes a constant supply of red cells, white blood cells and platelets. The body will replenish the elements given during a blood donation—some in a matter of hours and others in a matter of weeks.

Interval for Donation of Blood and Blood Components

The blood donated by donor will be again regenerated by his body. The plasma volume and platelets are replaced within

48 hours, granulocytes and other elements of plasma (proteins etc.) within 7 days, red blood cells in 56 days and iron lost is replaced in 8 weeks. Hence he can donate whole blood every 12 weeks (3 months). Plasmapheresis can be done at an interval of 48 hours. Donor can undergo platelet apheresis at an interval of 48 hours, twice in a week and 24 times in a year.

Voluntary donor is healthy and the blood donated is again regenerated in body. One unit of blood can save not one patient but three–four patients as it is separated into components like packed red blood cells, plasma, platelets, granulocytes and cryoprecipitate.

Blood donation is superior of all donations. The healthy and repeat donors are great asset of the blood bank which is doing human service to the mankind.

BLOOD DONATION

At the time blood donation Questionnaire for donors is provided and purpose of this is:

- To find out, if the donor is having any transmissible diseases. Transfusion transmitted diseases (TTDs) are deferrals, some are permanent and some temporary.

  Thus, screening of blood for infectious diseases is essential.
- The aim of blood transfusion is to do good to the patient.

Testing at Blood Bank for Transfusion Transmissible Infections (TTIs)

As per the rules of Indian Government (Drug Control Act) and National Aids Prevention and Control (NACO) policy, testing of every unit of blood is mandatory and blood collected is screened using highest quality of screening tests for TTIs/TTDs.

The donor is asked for any signs and symptoms of AIDS and high risk activities, foreign travel, donation risks, tests done on their blood and window periods of infections are evaluated.

Donors must document accurate information, and should understand the donation process and blood testing, and that blood donation is voluntary with informed decision.

Do not donate blood to be tested for a HIV/AIDS, hepatitis or any other infectious disease.

Counseling for Reactive Donors

If a blood sample tests positive for any TTI, then:
- Only the donor is informed, counseled and encouraged for further testing.
- A pre- and post-counseling of the donors is done by the doctors at the center.
- Donors who are HIV sero-reactive are referred to voluntary counseling and testing center (VCTC) or integrated counseling and testing center (ICTC) for post-donation counseling.
- For TTI other than HIV, the donor is informed about the positive status and is advised accordingly.

HIV Positive Patients

When the donor is found to be positive for HIV, following instructions have to be followed.
- Consult a clinician experienced in treating HIV/AIDS.
- Protect sex partner(s) from HIV by following safe-sex guidelines.
- Inform sex partner(s) who may also be infected.
- Do not share needles/blades/sharps contaminated with blood.
- Get psychological support from a counselor and/or join a support group for people with HIV.

Note: For more information refer to topic on TTDs.

Types of Blood Donors

There are different types of blood donors:
- Voluntary donors
- Replacement donors
- Autologous donors

Voluntary donor is one who donates blood for storage at a blood blank for transfusion to an unknown recipient.
- A greater percentage of better quality of blood comes from voluntary donors.
- These donors are very important because the incidence of blood transmitted infections is much less in blood drawn from these volunteers.

Replacement donor is a person, often a family member, donates blood for transfusion to a specific individual.

- The donor is selected by the recipient.
- Since there is pressure to donate, they may give blood even if there is risk behavior.

Autologous donor is a person who donates blood to be stored and is transfused back to himself/herself at a later stage, usually during and/or after surgery. **For details, please refer to Chapters on "Autologous blood transfusion" and "Blood substitutes"**.

Directed donation: When a person, often a family member, donates blood for transfusion to a specific individual, is called directed donation. This is only possible when the donor's blood type and other factors match the person needing the transfusion. Directed donations are relatively rare.

Directed Donation Procedure

A directed donation is a donation made for a specific recipient. Through directed donations, recipients can receive blood from family members and friends. Some recipients may feel more comfortable selecting their own donors. Directed donations may not be appropriate for emergency procedures since it takes time to fully test and process each unit of blood. If a physician recommends and/or a patient prefers to receive directed donations, blood bank can make every effort to collect, test, process, and distribute the blood units to the hospital for surgery.

It is the patient/recipient's responsibility, or they may select a representative to schedule directed donation appointments and ensure that these recruited donors keep their appointments. Directed donations are made by appointment only. Before donating, directed donors and recipients must follow a protocol.

1. Patients must obtain a prescription from their physician. It must include the patient's name, type and screen for directed donation, type and amount of blood product(s), date required, and hospital where the blood product(s) should be sent.

2. Donors can call the blood bank to schedule the directed donation. Patient's blood type should be known. If the patient does not know his or her blood type, a typing will be ordered by a physician, which can be performed at the blood bank or at its affiliated laboratory.

3. Patients need to recruit family members and friends for the required number of blood products needed. It is important to recruit extra donors since some of the selected donors may not have a compatible blood type, or may be not eligible to donate.

All directed donors must meet the same strict regulatory requirements for the general blood supply. Directed donors must also meet the same criteria as general blood donors regarding prior health history and should not have high-risk activities. Directed donors will be deferred from giving blood based upon the standard regulatory requirements for blood donation.

If directed donations meet all the safety requirements and for some reason (such as a change in the date of surgery) when blood cannot be used for the intended patients, these units of blood may be used for other patients.

Advantages and Disadvantages

There are **no medical advantages** to directed donation blood. It may seem safer to families for their infant/patient to receive blood from someone that they know. However, prevalence rate of infectious diseases is not necessarily lower in directed donors when compared with voluntary donors.

Donation from a husband to his wife during child bearing age is discouraged, to avoid likely pre-sensitisation.

Directed donations have risk of graft-versus-host disease (GvHD), which is sometimes seen in donations from blood relatives.

Delay

A directed donation must be co-ordinated by the patient and the donor of their specific choice, blood needs to be collected at the blood bank and further blood bank requires about

5–7 days to process the donated blood. Whereas blood previously received from voluntary donors is available to the patient right away.

Cost

Directed donations are costlier than the usual blood given by voluntary blood donations.

The American Red Cross has given permission for directed blood donation.

CRITERIA FOR DONOR SELECTION

Age: 18–65 years.

Minimum body weight: 45 kg.

A person can donate 8 mL/kg body weight (up to 450 mL every three months).

Haemoglobin (Hb): 12.5 gm% or above or Hct equal to more than 38%. Hb can be estimated by spectrophotometric or other methods. The haemoglobin is estimated by specific gravity method is mentioned here. Known specific gravity of blood that corresponds to the minimum acceptable haemoglobin level, necessary for safe blood donation is necessary. To know this, a drop of donor's red cells is dropped into the solution of copper sulphate. **The copper sulphate used to determine the donor acceptability has a specific gravity of 1.054 which is equal to the weight of a red cells with Hb of 12.5 gm/dL.** If the donor's haemoglobin is at acceptable minimum level, the specific gravity of donor's red cells is the same as the specific gravity

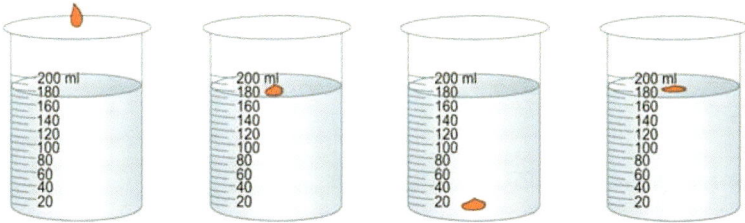

Fig. 2.1: Haemoglobin estimation by copper sulphate method

of copper sulphate. The drop of blood in the solution should stay in the centre for approximately for 15 seconds and then slowly sink to the bottom. If the Hb level is greater than the required level, the drop falls in the solution before 15 seconds. It the Hb level lower than required level, the drop of blood does not fall during the required 15 seconds. A decision on the donor's acceptability, can be made on the Hb content which can be easily made on this simple procedure.

Preparation of copper sulphate solution of specific gravity 1.054:

1. Dissolve 159.63 gm of pure dried crystals of copper sulphate ($CuSO_4.5H_2O$) and make the volume to 1000 mL at 25°C. This is stock solution. The specific gravity of this is 1.100.
2. Prepare working solution with specific gravity of 1.054 by adding 52 mL of stock solution and 48 mL of distilled water. This solution is stored at room temperature in tightly capped containers.

Donor Screening

Involves registration, consent of the donor, demographic information, medical history, limited physical examination and simple laboratory tests.

Demographic information: It should be complete and correct so that the donor can be informed of any laboratory testing abnormality.

1. Donor's full name
2. Father's/Husband's name
3. Age
4. Gender
5. Phone number
6. Residential address

Medical history:

1. History of any long-term illness.
2. Any medication if patient is taking.
3. Allergy to any substance/medication, etc.

Physical examination: A qualified practitioner of medicine or Blood Bank Officer will examine for the following:

- **General appearance:** A donor should be healthy.
- **Pulse:** 60–100 beats/minute.
- **Temperature:** 37°C.
- **Blood pressure:**
  - *Systolic pressure:* 100–140 mm of Hg
  - *Diastolic pressure:* 60–90 mm of Hg.
- Respiratory, cardiovascular, gastrointestinal, etc. systems should be normal and no problems should be detected by a rapid physical examination.

Informed consent: If the donor has successfully passed the history, physical examination, prior to donation, informed consent is required.

Laboratory tests: Following are the tests done on the unit of blood donated.

1. Haemoglobin estimation
2. Blood grouping and crossmatching
3. Screening for unwanted antibodies
4. Screening for transfusion transmissible infections: Indian Government regulatory authorities for blood bank recommends following 5 tests to be mandatory. These are mentioned below.
   - HIV 1 and 2
   - Hepatitis B
   - Hepatitis C
   - Syphilis
   - Malaria

Tests must be performed at each donation regardless of number of earlier donations.

Blood is not collected on the following occasions and depending upon the conditions they can be temporary deferral or permanent deferral.

Temporary deferrals are deferred temporarily on the following occasions: Hb <12.5 gm %, body weight <45 kg and if blood donated within last 3 months.

As an occupational hazard aircrews, drivers of long-distance heavy-duty vehicles and construction workers on high buildings are advised not to give blood within 12 hours of going on duty.

Respiratory infection

Cold, flu, cough, sore throat or acute sinusitis	Defer until all symptoms subside and temperature normal
Chronic sinusitis	No deferral unless using antibiotics
Asthmatic attack	1 week after last attack if chest is clear
Asthmatics on steroids	Defer

Pregnancy and abortion

Pregnancy or recently delivered	Defer for 6 months after delivery
Abortion	Defer for 6 months after abortion
Breast feeding	12 months after delivery

Women during menstrual cycle	Defer during menstrual cycle

Surgical procedures

Major surgery	12 months after recovery
Minor surgery	3 months after recovery
Open heart surgery including by-pass surgery	Permanently defer
Cancer surgery	Permanently defer
Localized skin cancer that was removed	Defer for 6 months after removal
Tooth extraction or dental manipulation	Defer for 3 days
Dental surgery under anesthesia	Defer for 1 month

Alcohol beverages	Defer if taken within 24 hr

Heart disease

Has any active symptom (chest pain, shortness of breath, swelling of feet)	Permanently defer
Restricted activity	Permanently defer
Cardiac medication (digitalis, nitroglycerine)	Permanently defer

Cardiovascular disease

Myocardial infarction	Permanently defer
Coronary artery disease	Permanently defer
Angina pectoris	Permanently defer
Rheumatic heart disease with residual damage	Permanently defer

Seizures

Convulsion and epilepsy	Permanently defer
Endocrinal disorders	Permanently defer

Infectious disease

Donors should be free from infectious diseases known to be transmissible by blood, so far as can be determined by usual examination and history.

Viral hepatitis

Has had hepatitis (jaundice other than hepatitis A, positive test for hepatitis B (HBsAg), hepatitis C (HCV))	Permanently defer
Exposure to possibility of hepatitis by tattoos, acupuncture or body piercing	Defer for 12 months
Worked in renal dialysis	Defer for 12 months
Received transfusion of blood and its component	Defer for 12 months
Close contact with individual suffering with hepatitis	Defer for 12 months

Jaundice

Has ever had jaundice associated with

Rh disease	No deferral
Gall stone	No deferral
Infectious mononucleosis (If no hepatitis)	Accept after 6 months

HIV infection/AIDS

High risk group for HIV infection	Permanently defer
HIV positive person	Permanently defer
Donor having symptoms of AIDS	Permanently defer
IV drug abusers	Permanently defer

Malaria

History of malaria in endemic area but duly treated and free from any symptoms	Accepted 3 years after treatment
Travel to endemic area	Defer for 1 year

Syphilis

Genital sores or generalized skin rashes	Defer for 12 months after rashes disappear and completion of therapy
Gonorrhea	12 months deferral after completion of therapy

Tuberculosis	Defer for 5 years after successful completion of treatment
Fever	
Had prolonged or rheumatic fever	Defer till fully recovered and off medication
Kidney disease	
Acute infection of kidney	Defer for 6 months after cessation or acute infection of bladder
Chronic kidney disease/failure	Permanently defer
Digestive system	
Stomach ulcer with symptoms or with recurrent bleeding	Permanently defer
Chronic liver disease/failure	Permanently defer

Medication

If donor is taking some medicine it may not be in his/her own interest to donate blood and may also affect the patient/recipient who would receive the blood.

Medicines	Accepted/Deferred
Oral contraceptive	Accepted
Analgesics	Accepted
Vitamins	Accepted
Mild sedative and tranquillizers	Accepted
Salicylates (Aspirin) taken in last three days	Not accepted if blood to be used for preparing platelets
Isotretinoin (Accutane) used for acne	Defer for 1 month after the last dose
Finasteride (i.e. Proscar) used to treat benign prostatic hyperplasia	Defer for 1 month after the last dose
Oral anti-diabetic drugs with no vascular complication	Acceptable
Diabetics on insulin	Defer while taking the drug
Antibiotics (oral)	Defer for 3 days and till symptom free
Antibiotics (injection)	Defer for 4 days and till symptom free/after the last injection
Cortisone	Defer for 7 days after the last dose
Medicine to treat hypercholesterolemia	Accepted

Donors taking following medicines are permanently rejected:

Anti-arrhythmics	Immunosuppressive drugs
Anticonvulsions	Pituitary growth hormones of human origin
Anticoagulants	Sedatives or tranquillisers in high dose
Antithyroid drugs	Vasodilators
Cytotoxic drugs	Etretinate to treat psoriasis. It is teratogenic.
Digitalis	Drugs for Parkinson's disease
Dilantin	

Vaccination and Deferral

No deferral	Two weeks deferral	Four weeks deferral	One year deferral
Tetanus	Smallpox	Anti-tetanus serum	Anti-rabies vaccination
Typhoid	Polio	Anti-venom serum	Hepatitis B immuno-globulin (HBIG)
Cholera	Measles	Anti-gas gangrene serum	Gammaglobulin
Diphtheria	Mumps	Rubella	
	Yellow fever		

Other conditions requiring permanent deferral are:

No person shall donate blood and no blood bank shall draw blood from person, suffering from any of the disease mentioned below, namely:

- Cancer
- Abnormal bleeding tendencies
- Unexpected weight loss
- Polycythemia vera
- Leprosy
- Schizophrenia
- Severe allergic disorders

Instructions to the Donor

The donor is instructed to have breakfast and then asked to donate blood. He has to feel well and be relaxed.

He is advised for the following, as post-donation instructions:

- Take more fluids for 24 hr after blood donation.
- Volume wise recovery of blood occurs in 48 hr after blood donation.
- No specific bed rest is required during post-donation period, general rest is advised.
- Donor is advised not to lift heavy articles or do vigorous exercises for 24 hr
- He is advised not to smoke for ½ an hr after donation.

Rarely there can be donor reactions and these needs to be managed

The reactions can categorized as follows:

Mild reactions:

- Symptoms: Nervousness, pallor, sweating, thready pulse, nausea, vomiting.
- Management: Stop donation.
  Immediately raise donor's feet by 45 degrees.

Moderate reactions:

- Symptoms: Increased period of unconsciousness, decreased pulse rate, continuous fall in blood pressure.
- Management: Stop donation, administer oxygen and separate the donor from the general area by using a screen.

Severe reactions:

- Symptoms: Convulsions.
- Management: Prevent donor from injuring himself/herself.

Emergency Drugs

The following emergency drugs must be available at the donation site:

Glucose powder

Tablets

- Paracetamol
- Diclofenac sodium

Injections
- Dexamethasone
- Diclofenac sodium
- Chlorpheniramine maleate
- Calcium gluconate
- Adrenaline
- IV fluids

Important Days

14th June: World Blood Donor's Day.

1st October: National Blood Donation Day.

Blood is donated on the birthday celebrations of important national and local leaders.

Donor Health Screening, Donor Suitability Evaluation, Phlebotomy, Post-Donation Care and Adverse Donor Reactions

The blood transfusion centers should ensure the following:

1. The donor is safe and will not suffer from any adverse reactions as a result of blood donation.
2. Also, the blood transfusion center should ensure that, the donated unit will not cause any adverse consequences for the recipient.

DONOR SCREENING

In order to provide safety to the donor and also to the recipient with quality blood, donor health screening is very essential.

Many organizations use photographic identification of the donors for accurate identification and this can prevent early whole blood donation, i.e. before three months.

After registration, the blood donor is provided with explanatory information about the blood donation process. This covers the screening process, phlebotomy, self-deferral and donor confidentiality.

The donor is counseled regarding donor criteria for donor selection.

After the information and counseling procedure, the donor answers questionnaire designed to safeguard the donor himself and also the recipient who receives his blood. The donor has to answer the "Yes or No" questions.

The donor signs the consent form. He agrees for his unit of blood being tested for transfusion transmitted infections and being informed about the positive results.

DONOR HEALTH HISTORY AND DONOR SAFETY

The blood donors must be in good health. After the donation process, the volume lost is mostly replaced within a few hours and completely within 48–72 hours. Iron stores and red cells are replaced within 7–8 weeks. Thus, blood donation is limited to once in three months to allow the donor with sufficient time for absorption of dietary iron to prevent himself from developing iron deficiency anaemia.

Open-ended questions may be asked to know the overall health of the donor. Specific questions relating to cardiac disease, lung disease, liver disease, blood disease, pregnancy and history of cancer may be asked. Donors with medical history are not permitted to donate.

Donors on medication may indicate some medical problem with donor, e.g. a donor on antibiotics signifies infection in a donor or some medication of donor can affect the recipient, e.g. donors on aspirin can have anti-platelet effect.

Weight of the donor is important for calculation of blood to be drawn. Standards allow donation of 13% of circulating volume of blood. Thus, a person who weighs 50 kg can donate 450 mL of whole blood and a person who weighs 45 kg can donate 350 mL of blood.

Age of the donor must be 18 years or more (some countries like USA and Scotland age of 17 years is acceptable).

DONOR HEALTH HISTORY AND RECIPIENT SAFETY

The most of the questions asked are relating to protect the recipient from infectious diseases originating from the donor.

The blood borne diseases such as:
1. HIV-1 and HIV-2
2. Viral hepatitis B and C
3. Malaria
4. Syphilis
5. Babesiosis
6. Chagas disease
7. West Nile virus (WNV)

Some of these are permanently deferred and some temporarily deferred for prescribed period of time after treatment.

Note: Refer to topic on TTDs.

DONOR PHYSICAL EXAMINATION

Donor physical examination is to evaluate donor's vital signs which are checked before donation.

1. Pulse rate and rhythm
2. Blood pressure
3. Temperature
4. Venipuncture sites

Individuals with a fever, high blood pressure (generally higher than 180/100 mm of Hg), very high or very low heart rate or an irregular heart beat are not permitted to donate blood.

The donor's pulse of 60 to 100/min. is acceptable. Athletic donors with pulse of 50/minute is acceptable.

The donor's blood pressure of systolic 100–140 mm of Hg and diastolic of 60 to 90 mm of Hg is arbitrarily acceptable.

Donor's temperature of more than normal is not acceptable. Elevated temperature signifies potential source of infectious agent to a recipient.

Inspect the arm for infections, scars and venipuncture site for any signs of drug abuse.

To make sure that blood is not drawn from anaemic donor, the haemoglobin of the donor has to be 12.5 gm% or more and haematocrit has to be 38%.

CONFIDENTIAL UNIT EXCLUSION (CUE)

Some of the donors donate under pressure of their peers, friends or relatives. In such occasions, in some countries an opportunity is given to the donors to exclude units confidentially. A confidential unit exclusion form is given to the donors and such units are not used for transfusion and are discarded. Some countries do not follow this CUE.

Steps for Donor Suitability Evaluation

The steps of donor suitability evaluation are as follows.

PHLEBOTOMY

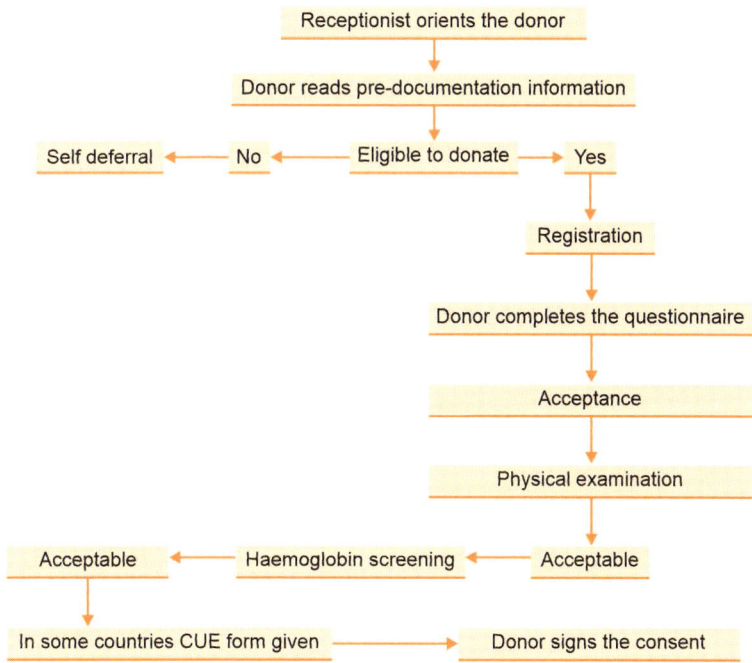

The phlebotomist has to follow the following guidelines of WHO best practices in phlebotomy[3] for drawing blood:

Step 1. Identify donor and label blood collection bag and test tubes

- Ask the donor to state his/her full name.
- Ensure that:
  The blood collection bag is of the correct type;
  The labels on the blood collection bag and all its satellite bags, sample tubes and donor records have the correct donor name and number;
  The information on the labels matches with the donor's information.

Step 2. Select the vein

- Select a large, firm vein, preferably in the antecubital fossa, from an area free from skin lesions or scars.
- Apply a tourniquet or blood pressure cuff inflated to 40–60 mm Hg, to make the vein more prominent.
- Ask the donor to open and close the fist a few times.

Step 3. Disinfect the skin

- If the site selected for venipuncture is visibly dirty, wash the area with soap and water, and then wipe it dry.
- **One-step procedure (recommended—takes about one minute):** Use a product combining 2% chlorhexidine gluconate in 70% isopropyl alcohol; cover the whole area and ensure that the skin area is in contact with the disinfectant for **at least** 30 seconds; allow the area to dry **completely**.
- Two-step procedure (if chlorhexidine gluconate in 70% isopropyl alcohol is not available, use the following procedure—takes about two minutes):
  Step 1—use 70% isopropyl alcohol; cover the whole area and ensure that the skin area is in contact with the disinfectant for **at least** 30 seconds; allow the area to dry **completely**.
  Step 2—use tincture iodine (more effective than povidine iodine) or chlorhexidine (2%); cover the whole area and ensure that the skin area is in contact with the disinfectant for **at least** 30 seconds; allow the area to dry **completely.**
- Whichever procedure is used, DO NOT touch the venipuncture site once the skin has been disinfected.

Step 4. Perform the venipuncture

Perform venipuncture using a smooth, clean entry with the needle and the needle should be cut off at the end of the procedure rather than re-capped.

- Ask the donor to open and close the fist slowly every 10–12 seconds during collection.

Step 5. Monitor the donor and the donated unit

- Closely monitor the donor and the venipuncture site throughout the donation process—look for sweating, pallor or complaints of feeling faint that may precede fainting; development of a haematoma at the venipuncture site; changes in blood flow that may indicate the needle has moved out of the vein, and needs to be repositioned.

- About every 30 seconds during the donation, mix the collected blood gently with the anticoagulant, either manually or by keeping on continuous mechanical mixing instrument.
- Remove the tourniquet or release blood pressure cuff after the procedure is complete.

Step 6. Remove the needle and collect samples

- Collect blood samples for laboratory testing.
- Cut off the needle using a sterile pair of scissors.

POST-DONATION CARE

After a blood donation, following care has to be taken and some instructions have to be given

1. Donor care: After the blood has been collected:
   - Ask the donor to remain in the chair and relax for a few minutes (10 minutes);
   - Inspect the venipuncture site; if it is not bleeding, apply a bandage to the site; if it is bleeding, apply further pressure and raise the arm.
   - Ask the donor to sit up slowly and ask how the person is feeling.
   - Before the donor leaves the donation room, ensure that the person can stand up without dizziness and without drop in blood pressure.
   - If donor feels dizzy, ask him/her to lie down.
   - If fainting and bleeding persists, see that the physician attends him/her.
   - Inform the staff immediately if any unexpected reactions occur.
   - Offer the donor some refreshments: Donor should eat and drink before leaving the place.
   - Ask the donor to drink more fluids for next four hours.
   - Ask the donor not to smoke or ride/drive vehicle for at least one and a half hours after blood donation.

2. Blood unit and samples
   - Transfer the blood unit to a proper storage container according to the blood centre requirements and the product.
   - Ensure that collected blood samples are stored and delivered to the laboratory with completed documentation, at the recommended temperature, and in a leak-proof, closed container.

ADVERSE DONOR REACTIONS

Although the donation process is safe and uncomplicated, occasional adverse donor reactions may occur. These can be reduced or avoided by proper donor selection and care. Donors who suffer adverse donor reactions, they may not or they are less likely to donate again.

Haematoma formation occurs in 2–3% of the donors. Causes are:

1. Poor or failed venipuncture
2. Needle puncturing the vein twice during the donation
3. Inadequate pressure after the donation

In such instances:

1. Apply pressure and a firm bandage
2. Reassure the donor
3. Give relevant contact information to the donor, in case the donor has any further inquiries.
4. Local application of thrombophobe ointment may be advised.

Vasovagal episodes and soft tissue injuries (bruises and haematomas at the venipuncture site) are the most common donor reactions. These occur in 1% of the donors. This is due to hypothalamic response resulting in bradycardia, vomiting, sweating, arterial dilatation and a low blood pressure. The majority of these are minor and donor recovers immediately. If fainting occurs after completion of the donation procedure advise rest, elevate foot end, monitor pulse and blood pressure and give plenty of oral fluids. For such donors reassurance should be provided so as to again donate. If symptoms occur during bleeding procedure, stop bleeding and monitor the vitals. Provide foot end elevation. Fluids may be given orally or IV, if necessary. With severe reactions, donor should not donate again. Young and first time donor are likely to have adverse donor reactions.

Causes for vasovagal episodes are:
1. Anxiety
2. Lowered blood volume and other associated causes:
   - Hypoglycaemia
   - Lack of fluids
   - Poor sleep
3. Atmosphere in donation room (hot or humid)

Signs and symptoms for vasovagal episodes are:
1. Staring
2. Sighing
3. Pallor or sweating
4. Slow pulse
5. Drop in blood pressure
6. Vomiting
7. Loss of consciousness (occasionally)
8. Convulsions (occasionally)

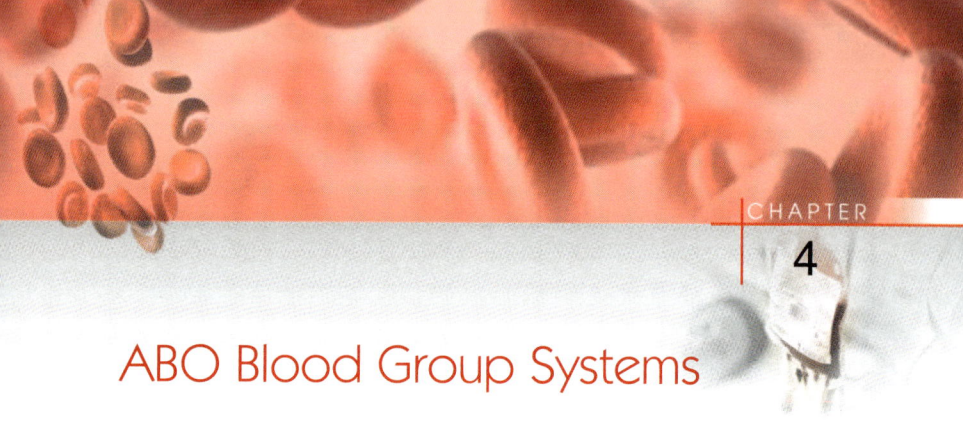

4

ABO Blood Group Systems

The red cells have antigens on their surface. The importance of red cell antigens is manifold. Since the work of Landsteiner in early 1900s, it has been recognized that knowledge and understanding of blood groups is essential for transfusion therapy.

HISTORY OF BLOOD GROUPS

The major events in history of blood transfusion are given as follows:

1900 Karl Landsteiner (Austrian physician), discovered **A, B and O**.

AB blood group was discovered in the year 1902 by **A Decastello and A Sturli.**

1939/40: The Rh blood group system was discovered by **Karl Landsteiner, Alex Wiener, Philip Levine and RE Stetson.**

1945: Coombs, Mourant and Race discovered **anti-human globulin** (Coombs' test) for **incomplete antibodies**.

However, the efforts to discover blood groups were started much earlier. The events are given below:

1628: English physician **William Harvey** discovered the circulation of blood.

1665–67: Physician Richard Lower (England) and Jean-Baptiste Denis (France) recorded successful blood transfusion in animals and report transfusions from lambs to humans.

After this, transfusing the blood of animals to humans became prohibited by law, delaying the advances in transfusion medicine for about 150 years.

1795: In Philadelphia, an American physician, Philip Syng Physick, claimed to perform the first human blood transfusion, although he did not publish this information.

1818: James Blundell, a British obstetrician, transfused human blood to a case of postpartum haemorrhage. During 1825 to 1830, he did 10 transfusions, five of these were beneficial to the patients, and he published these results.

1840: Samuel Armstrong Lane and Blundell, undertook first successful whole blood transfusion to treat a case of haemophilia.

In 1900 and 1902 the major milestone was discovery of A, B, O and AB blood groups as stated above.

Landsteiner received the Nobel Prize for Medicine for this discovery in 1930.

In **1907** Hektoen suggested that the safety of transfusion might be improved by crossmatching.

In **1912** Roger Lee (physician) from Massachusetts General Hospital coined "Universal Donor" **and** "Universal Recipient".

In **1939/40** another major blood group 'Rh' was discovered followed by **1945,** a test to detect **'Incomplete Antibodies'** by using **anti-human globulin (Coombs' test)** was established.

History of other rare blood groups:

MNS system was discovered in the year 1927.

P Blood group system was also discovered in the same year as MNS system, i.e. 1927.

Kell blood group was discovered in the year 1946 which was named after Mrs. Kellner, mother of the first child to be affected with HDN.

Duffy in 1950, Mr. Duffy was a hemophilia patient.

Kidd blood group was named after Mrs. Kidd whose serum contained the antibody and antigen was named 'JK' after woman's child **John Kidd,** who suffered **HDN.**

Bombay blood group was discovered by **Dr YM Bhende** and **colleagues** in the year 1952.

RED CELL BLOOD GROUP SYSTEMS

In routine practice, it is necessary to determine the compatibility of certain red cell antigens between the donor and the recipient. Also understanding of other blood group systems such as Kell, may be associated with both functional and morphological changes in the red cells. Study of inheritance of blood group antigens provides a greater understanding of the mechanism of gene expression.

Amongst these, the two most important blood groups in blood transfusion are:

- ABO system
- Rh system

International Society of Blood Transfusion (ISBT) has instituted a numerical system of nomenclature to standardize red cell blood grouping terminology. According to ISBT (2004) around 30 blood group systems are known.

Different blood group systems

Number	Name	Abbreviation
001	ABO	ABO
002	MNSs	MNSs
003	P	P
004	Rh	Rh
005	Lutheran	LU
006	Kell	KEL
007	Lewis	LE
008	Duffy	FY
009	Kidd	JK
010	Diego	DI
011	Cartwright	YT
012	XG	XG
013	Scianna	SC
014	Dombrock	DO
015	Colton	CO
016	Landsteiner-Wiener	LW
017	Chido/Rodgers	CH/RG
018	Hb	H
019	Kx	XK
020	Geribich	GH

(Contd.)

Number	Name	Abbreviation
021	Cromer	CROM
022	Knops	KN
023	Indian	IN
024	Ok	OK
025	Raph	RAPH
026	John Milton Hagan	JMH
027	I	I
028	Gloside	GLOB
029	GIL	GIL
030	RHAG	RHAG

Indian blood group is named after the country, 4% Indians from Bombay express this blood group. The antigen is encoded by the CD44 gene located on chromosome 11p13.

It has two variants as shown below:

- IN a   IgG Antibodies   HDN No   No HTR
- IN b   IgG Antibodies   HDN No   Rare HTR

Importance of ABO Grouping

- ABO compatibility between donor cells and patient serum is the essential foundation of pre-transfusion testing.
- It is the blood group system with **expected antibodies.**
- Whether they are **IgG or IgM, ABO** antibodies can activate complement readily.
- This means that **incompatibilities** can cause **life-threatening situations** (transfusion reactions).
- It is so important that a mistake in grouping and transfusing can lead to grave complications.

ABO System

- It is based on the presence of two antigens on the wall of RBCs: **A antigen and B antigen**. These antigens are formed from a basic antigen called H antigen which is present in all individuals with rare exception.
- ABO blood groups: A, B, AB and O.
- ABO system **obeys Landsteiner Laws** with regard to **antigen and antibodies**.

Landsteiner Laws

Law 1: If an individual has an antigen on the wall of red cell, the corresponding antibody should not be present in plasma.

Law 2: If an individual has an antibody in the plasma, the corresponding antigen should not be present on the wall of red cell.

Blood Group Antigens

- The antigenic determinants or epitopes are small portions of molecules recognised by antibodies. **ABO antigens are carbohydrate in nature.** They are oligosaccharide chains anchored to glycoproteins or glycolipids of the RBC membrane.
- They are **highly immunogenic**. A and B antigens **differ in only the terminal sugar**. There is terminal sugar **N-acetyl galactosamine in A group** and terminal sugar **galactose in B group**.
- There is no A or B antigen in O blood group. There is **absence of terminal sugars in O phenotype.**

Antibodies

- In ABO system there are natural antibodies. They are present in the serum/plasma. They are **IgM type** and have high molecular weight and hence cannot pass through the placenta.
- These antibodies react well at 4°C, room temperature or at 37°C.
- Sometimes IgG anti-antibodies may be produced in O blood group patients and sometimes by A2 blood group patients, which can cause haemolytic transfusion reactions and haemolytic disease of newborn.
- Antibodies of ABO blood group system react at a wide temperature range and potentially haemolytic at 37 degree C. Group O donors should always be screened for IgG (hyperimmune) anti-A and anti-B antibodies which may cause haemolysis, when group O whole blood is transfused to recipients of A or B blood groups. These dangerous O donors should be used for O recipients only or should be used as packed red cells.

TABLE 4.1: ABO blood groups: Antigens, antibodies and frequency of occurrence			
Name of blood group	*Antigens*	*Antibodies*	*Frequency of occurrence*
AB	A, B	None	3%
A	A	Anti-B	42%
B	B	Anti-A	8%
O	None	Anti-A, Anti-B	47%

The frequency of occurrence of ABO blood groups varies from country to country and region to region.

Genetics

- The genes for ABO system are at three separate loci (ABO, Hh and Se) which control the occurrence and location of the A and B antigens.
- Three common alleles for ABO (A, B, and O) are located at the ABO locus on **chromosome 9.** The genes occupy **9q34.1-q34.2** has 7 exons and is of 18 kb. A and B genes differ in 7 nucleotides, difference is mainly in amino acids at 266 and 267 in exon 7.
- The A and B genes encode glycosyl transferase that produces A and B antigens, respectively.
- The red cells of O person lack **A and B antigens, but carry abundant amount of H antigen**, the precursor material on which A and B antigens are built.
- The genes for two loci, **Hh and Se (Secretor), are on the chromosome 19** and are closely linked.
- **H gene** (19q13.3) transmitted in **Mendelian Manner.** Each locus has two recognized alleles, one of which has no demonstrable product. The active allele at the H locus, H produces a glycosyl transferase that acts at the cellular level to form H antigen on which A or B are built.
- The Se gene is directly responsible for the expression of H antigen, which may then be modified to express A and B on the glycoproteins in epithelial secretions such as saliva. Eighty percent of the population are secretors. Secretors have inherited the Se gene and express H antigen, which can be converted to A and/or B if they also have the A and/or B gene.

Gene	Enzyme coded	Sugar added by enzyme
	TABLE 4.2: To show enzymes and sugars added in different blood groups	
A	N-acetyl galactosamyl transferase	N-acetyl galactosamine
B	Galactosyl transferase	Galactose
H	Fucosyl transferase	Fucose
O	Defective glycosyl transferase	None

H Antigen

- The H gene codes for an enzyme that adds the sugar fucose to the terminal sugar of a precursor substance (PS). The precursor substance (proteins and lipids) is formed on an oligosaccharide chain (the basic structure).

- The H antigen is the foundation upon which A and B antigens are built.

- A and B genes code for enzymes that add an immuno-dominant sugar to the H antigen. Immunodominant sugars are present at the terminal ends of the chains and confer the ABO antigen specificity.

- **Lectin from *Ulex europaeus* is source of anti-H and can detect H antigen**.

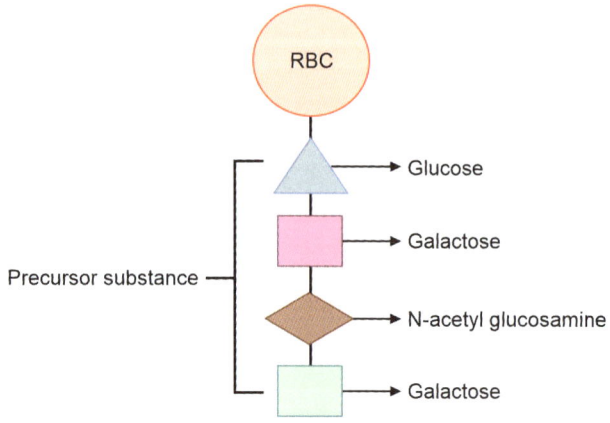

Fig. 4.1: RBC precursor substance

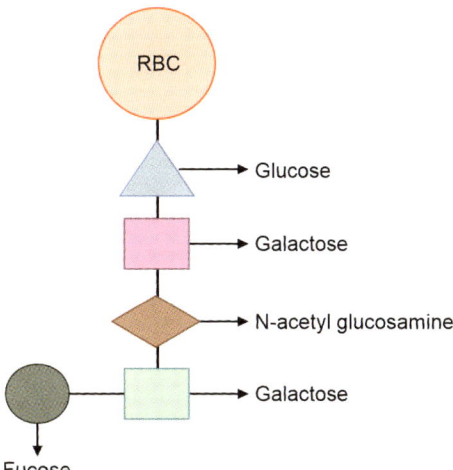

Fig. 4.2: Formation of H antigen on RBC precursor substance

A and B Antigens

The "Λ" gene codes for an enzyme (N-acetyl galactosaminyl transferase) that adds **N-acetyl galactosamine** to the terminal sugar of the H antigen.

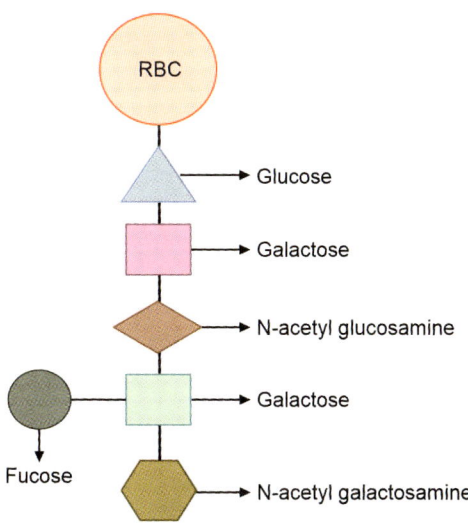

Fig. 4.3: Formation of A antigen with addition of N-acetyl galactosamine to H antigen.

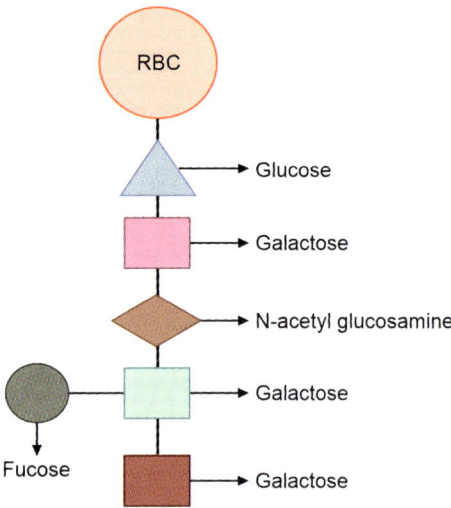

Fig. 4.4: Formation of B antigen with addition of galactose to H antigen

The "B" gene codes for an enzyme D-galactosyl transferase that adds **D-galactose** to the terminal sugar of the H antigen.

Association of Blood Groups with Diseases

'A' blood group is frequently associated with gastric carcinoma and 'O' blood group is frequent in peptic ulcer patients.

Universal Donors and Recipients

- The earlier concept of **'O' blood group as universal donor** and **AB blood group as universal recipient** does not hold good in recent years.
- 'O' blood group person has no antigens on the red cells but has anti-A and anti-B antibodies in the serum. When given to recipient, these antibodies can destroy some of the recipient's red cells. Hence, 'O' blood, better not to be given to A, B or AB persons. **However, washed 'O' red cells can be given.**
- Earlier notion of AB person as a universal recipient, as they have A and B antigen on the red cells does not hold good. A or B blood groups will have antibodies against AB blood group antigens and can destroy some red cells of the AB recipient. Hence A or B blood groups better not to be

transfused to AB blood group patient. However, AB plasma can be given to A, B or O persons as it does not have any antibodies. Hence, **washed O red cell packs** and **AB plasma** are **universal donors.**

Bombay Blood Group

- In this blood group the red cells lack H, A and B antigens. It was first discovered in Bombay (India) in 1952 by Dr YM Bhende and colleagues.
- Symbol Oh denotes the phenotype, on routine ABO typing tests **Bombay blood group** mimic those of group O persons.
- Oh serum contains strong anti-H, anti-A and anti-B antibodies.
- When serum from the Oh is tested against group O red cells, after immediate-spin strong agglutination and/or haemolysis occurs.

Note: For details refer to chapter on **"subgroups and weaker variants of A and B blood groups and Bombay phenotype".**

Para-Bombay Phenotypes

Para-Bombay phenotypes have a non-functional H gene but a normal Se gene and thus, will express A, B and H antigens in their plasma and secretions.

The sera of A_h and B_h people contain anti-H in addition to the expected anti-A or anti-B antibodies.

ABO Antigens in Secretions

- **Secretions** include body fluids like plasma, saliva, synovial fluid, etc.
- Blood group substances are soluble antigens (A, B, and H) that can be found in the secretions. This is controlled by the H and Se genes.
- The secretor gene consists of 2 alleles (Se and se).
- The **Se gene** is responsible for the expression of the **H antigen** on glycoprotein structures located in body secretions.
- If the Se allele is inherited as SeSe or Sese, the person is called a **"secretor"**. 80% of the population are secretors.

- **Secretors** express soluble forms of **the H antigen** in secretions that can then be converted to A or B antigens (by the transferases). Individuals who inherit the sese gene are called "nonsecretors". The se allele is amorph (nothing expressed).
- **sese** individuals do not convert antigen precursors to H antigen and has neither soluble H antigen nor soluble A or B antigens in body fluids.
- The **Se gene** codes for the presence of the **H antigen in secretions**, therefore the presence of A and/or B antigens in the secretions is contingent on the inheritance of the *Se* gene and the *H* gene.

ABO Discrepancy

- An ABO discrepancy is said to exist when forward and reverse typing do not agree.
- The patient's serum contains ABO antibodies not compatible with the antigens on red cells detected by forward grouping.
- A and B antigen expression can be weakened in acute leukemias especially the A blood group (acute myeloid leukemias) or some carcinomas (stomach or pancreas).

Note: For details refer to chapter on **errors and discrepancies in ABO typing.**

Rh System

- After A, B, H antigens, the D antigen of the Rh system has the most significant implications in transfusion practice.
- Patients with D antigen are said to be positive.
- The Rh system also contains other clinically significant antigens (C, E, c and e) and less significant antigens (variant, *cis* products and G antigens).
- IgG antibodies can be produced in Rh system with immunological sensitization.

Note: For details refer to the chapter on **Rh typing and weaker variants of Rh system.**

Other Important Blood Groups

MNSs System

- M and N alphabets are derived from the word IMMUNE and S from the name of place Sydney city where this blood group was discovered.
- There are two loci: M/N and S/s. The antigens are M, N, S, and s.
- Anti-M and anti-N are naturally occurring (IgM) antibodies.
- Anti-S and anti-s are IgG class antibodies as a result of pregnancy or transfusion.

P System

- This blood group was discovered by Landsteiner and Levine, the gene is located on chromosome **22q11.2**.
- P1 is the most common antigen which has variable strength of expression.
- **Anti-P1** may be naturally occurring.
- It is most often an **IgM antibody**.

Lutheran (Lu) System

- This system has a single locus on chromosome 19q13.32, has 19 antigens of which the antigens Lua and Lub are strong ones.
- The Lu(a) negative phenotype is very rare.
- Antibodies **to Lutheran antigens are IgG type.**
- The genes of the Lutheran group are linked to the genes responsible for the secretion of ABH substances.

Kell System

- This blood group has four antigens at two loci: K (Kell) and k (cellano), and Kpa and Kpb.
- The Kp(a+) phenotype and the Kp(a-b-) phenotype are both rare.
- The Knull phenotype K-k-Kp(a-b-) is associated with chronic granulomatous disease (CGD), an inherited defect in the bacterial phagocytosis of neutrophils.
- Antibodies to Kell system antigens are IgG, named after the family of the antibody producer Mrs. Kellner who suffered haemolytic transfusion reaction and her baby had haemolytic disease of newborn.

- **McLeod syndrome:** In 1961, Allen and co-workers found that one of their students, Mr. McLeod, had RBCs with weak expression of Kell antigens. He had lacked Kx protein which is important for expression of Kell antigen.
- These patients will have weak expression of Kell blood group antigens and have acanthocytes, haemolytic anaemia and elevated serum creatinine kinase. These patients have muscular and neurological defects.

Lewis System

- This system focuses on a single locus with two antigens, Le a and Le b on chromosome 19.
- These antigens do not form an integral part of the red cell membrane, but are soluble antigens which may be present in body fluids and secretions.
- They are adsorbed on to the surface of red cells if they are present in the plasma in sufficient amounts.
- There are only three phenotypes: Le(a-b-); Le(a+b-); and Le(a-b+). Lewis phenotypes may change during pregnancy.
- Lewis antibodies are IgM type.

Duffy System

- The Duffy system has single locus with two antigens Fy a and Fy b.
- The only rare phenotype is Fy(a-b-), which has a higher frequency in countries where there is a high incidence of *Plasmodium falciparum* malaria.
- This phenotype gives a degree of immunity to the disease because the malarial parasite requires Duffy antigens to enter the red cells.
- **Duffy antibodies** are almost **exclusively IgG type**.
- This system is named after the family of the antibody producer, Duffy.

Kidd (Jk) System

- The genes are on single locus, two-antigen system (Jka and Jkb). There are four possible phenotypes: Jk(a-b-); Jk(a+b-); Jk(a-b+); Jk(a+b+).

- Jk(a-b-) is a rare phenotype.
- Antibodies to the Kidd antigens are almost exclusively IgG.
- Incompatible transfusion or pregnancy can lead to the formation of antibodies to all these blood groups, if the recipient/mother lacks the relevant antigen.

LABORATORY TESTING: ABO BLOOD GROUPING

Forward Grouping

Reaction of **patient red blood cells** is tested with reagent anti-A and anti-B and anti-AB antiseras by the following methods:
- Slide method
- Tube technique
- Matrix gel card method

Slide method: Always confirm the results of slide with tube test.

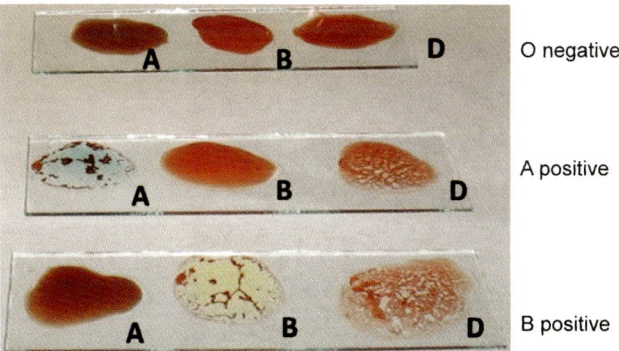

Fig. 4.5: Blood grouping by slide method

Procedure

Place 1 drop of anti-A and anti-B reagent separately on a labeled plane glass slide or concavity slide. Add 1 drop of saline diluted red cell suspension to each. Mix the cells and reagent with a slick or a glass rod using different ends. Tilt the slide and look for agglutination after 2 minutes at room temperature. Record the results.

Tube technique

- Prepare 2–5% suspension of RBCs.
- Take 3 test tubes.

1st test tube	2nd test tube	3rd test tube
1 drop of anti-A + 1 drop of cell suspension	1 drop of anti-B + 1 drop of cell suspension	1 drop of anti-A,B + 1 drop of cell suspension

Centrifuge at 1000 rpm × 1 minute.
Observe for agglutination.

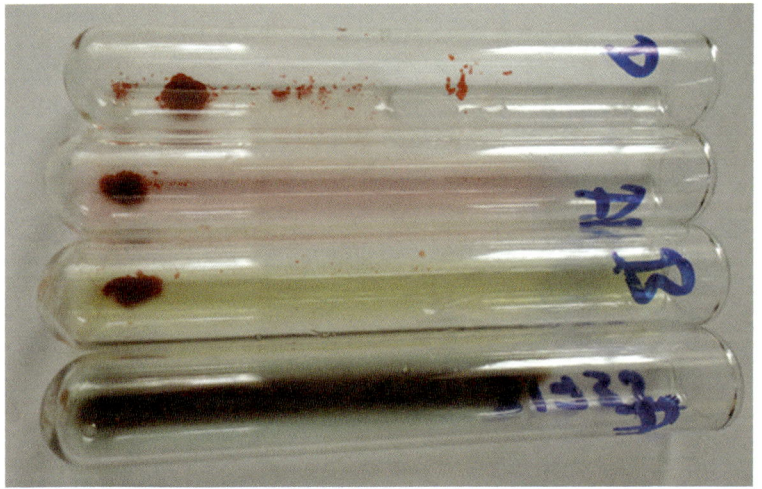

Fig. 4.6: ABO blood grouping and Rh typing by tube technique

Matrix gel system for ABO and Rh confirmation: Forward grouping

Matrix gel system has the following:
- Neutral gel in microtubes.
- Preservative—0.1% sodium azide.
- Store the gel cards at 4–25 degree C, do not freeze.
- Wash the cells twice and prepare cell suspension of 2–5%.
- Add 25 µl of cell suspension to all the tubes.
- Centrifuge 1200 rpm × 10 min.

- Observe for agglutination.
- Clear line on the matrix gel surface: Agglutination (positive).
- Compact cell button at the bottom: No agglutination (negative).

Reverse Grouping

Reaction of the patient's serum with known group A and group B cells is tested and the procedure is as given below.

- 50 µl of serum to A and B microtubes.
- 25 µl of known A cells and B cells.
- Allow the cards to incubate for 10 min at room temperature (18–25 degree C).
- Centrifuge at 1200 rpm × 10 min.
- Observe for agglutination.

ABO forward (cell) grouping reaction with result:

Sl No.	Anti-A	Anti-B	Blood group
1.	++++	Negative	A
2.	Negative	++++	B
3.	++++	++++	AB
4.	Negative	Negative	O

Reagents: Anti-A, anti-B, anti-AB

ABO reverse (serum) grouping reaction with result:

Sl No.	A cells	B cells	Blood group
1.	Negative	++++	A
2.	++++	Negative	B
3.	Negative	Negative	AB
4.	++++	++++	O

Reagent cells: Pooled A cells, B cells, O cells.

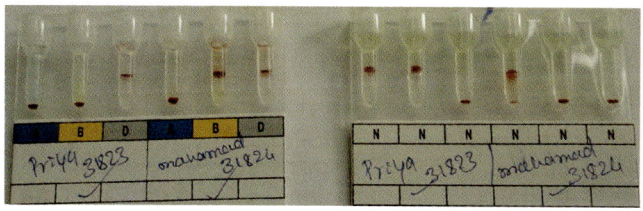

Fig. 4.7: Matrix gel card method, forward and reverse grouping

Strength of reaction	Comments
4+	Agglutinated red blood cells form a band at the top of the column
3+	Most agglutinated red blood cells remain in the upper half of gel column
2+	Agglutinated red blood cells are observed throughout the length of the column. A small botton of red blood cells may also be visible at the bottom of the gel column
1+	Most agglutinated red blood cells remain in the lower half of the column. A button of red blood cells may also be visible at the bottom of the gel column
±	Most agglutinated red blood cells remain in the lower third part of the column.
Negative (0)	All the red cells pass through and form a compact button at the bottom of the gel column
Mixed field agglutination	Agglutinated red blood cells form a band at the top of the gel or dispersed in the matrix and non-agglutinated red blood cells form a compact button at the bottom of the gel column
H	Hemolysis of red blood cells

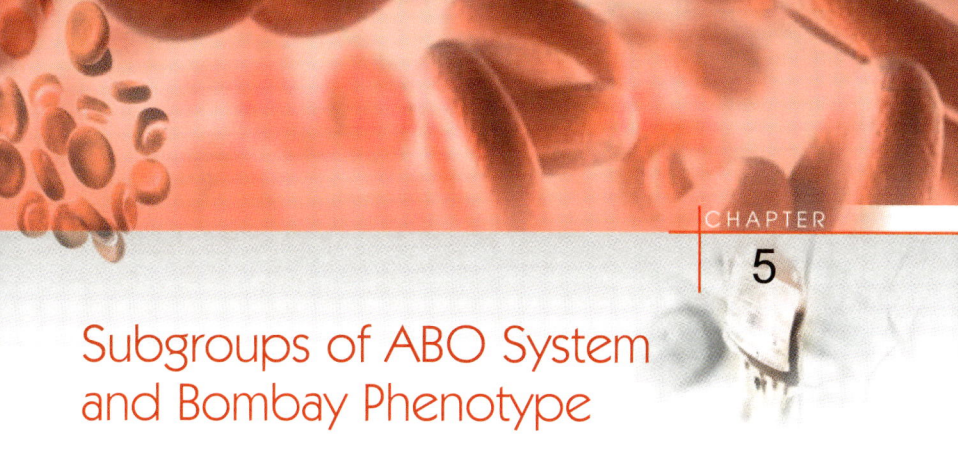

Subgroups of ABO System and Bombay Phenotype

For practical purposes, the ABO blood group is divided into A, B, AB and O blood groups. Only when problems arise subgroups are looked into and distinction of A and B subtypes is made.

SUBGROUPS OF ABO SYSTEM

There are many subgroups of ABO system. They are mentioned below:

Group A: The important subgroups of A are A1 and A2.

The other subgroups are: A_3, A_x, A_m, A_y A_{el}, Ae_{nd}, A_{bantu}, A_{finn}, and A_{int}.

The weaker variants are: A_2, A_3, A_x, A_m, $A_y A_{el}$, A_{end}, A_{bantu}, A_{finn}, and A_{int}.

Group B: The subgroups are: B, B_3, B_x, B_m, Bel, the weaker variants are: B_3, B_x, B_m, B_{el}.

Clinically Important Subgroups

The subgroups of blood group A having clinical importance are A_1 and A_2.

Serological differences between A1 and A2 are based on reactivity with human anti-A1 or anti-A1 lectin from *Dolichos biflorus*.

Amongst A blood group, 80% of population belongs to A1 blood group and about 20% belongs to A2 blood group.

55

About 1–8% of the A2 blood group individuals have anti-A1 antibodies.

Also about 22–35% of the A2B blood group individuals have anti-A1 antibodies.

A2 blood group has diminished enzyme activity and weak expression.

A2 if misdiagnosed as O blood group and when given to O blood group patients, the anti-A and anti-B antibodies present in the patient's serum will destroy the transfused blood.

BOMBAY PHENOTYPE (BOMBAY BLOOD GROUP)

Individuals with the rare Bombay phenotype (hh) do not express antigen H on their red blood cells. As H antigen serves as precursor for producing A and B antigens, the absence of H antigen means the individuals do not have A or B antigens as well (similar to O blood group). However, unlike O group, the H antigen is absent, hence the individuals produce isoantibodies to antigen H as well as to both A and B antigens. In case they receive blood from O blood group, the anti-H antibodies will bind to H antigen on RBC of donor blood and destroy the RBCs by complement-mediated lysis. **Therefore, Bombay phenotype can receive blood only from *hh* donors (Bombay blood group).**

Thus, in this blood group:
- The red cells lack H, A and B antigen.
- It was first discovered in Bombay in 1952 by Dr YM Bhende and colleagues.
- Symbol Oh denotes the phenotype, on routine ABO typing tests Bombay blood group mimic those of group O persons.
- Oh serum contains strong anti-H, anti-A and anti-B. When serum from the Oh is tested against group O red cells, after immediate-spin strong agglutination and/or haemolysis occurs.
- This blood group occurs 1 in 13000 population all over the world.

Para-Bombay Phenotypes

- Ah, Bh and ABh red cells lack serologically detectable H antigen but carry small amounts of A and/or B antigen, depending on the individual's genes at the ABO locus.

- Tests with anti-A or anti-B reagents may or may not give weak reactions but the cells are non-reactive with anti-H lectin or with anti-H serum from Oh persons.

- Para-Bombay phenotypes have a non-functional H gene but a normal Se gene and thus will express A, B and H antigens in their plasma and secretions.

- The sera of Ah and Bh people contain anti-H in addition to the expected anti-A or anti-B antibodies.

Rh Typing and Weaker Variants of Rh System

Discovery of D Antigen

The first human example of the antibody against the D antigen was reported in **1939 by Levin and Stetson.**

In 1940 Landsteiner and Wiener described an antibody obtained by immunizing guinea pigs and rabbits with the red cells of Rhesus monkey, which agglutinated approximately 85% of humans tested and the corresponding determinant was called.

Rh Factor

After A, B, O antigen, the D antigen of the Rh system has the most significant implications in transfusion practice.

The Rh system also contains other clinically significant antigens (C, E, c and e) and also less significant antigens (variant forms, *cis* products and G antigens).

Rh system is most complex genetically of all blood group types since it involves 45 different antigens on the surface of red cells. There are two possible alleles at each locus: c or C; d or D; and e or E.

- According to Fisher and Race system, there are 3 pairs of genetic alleles, namely Cc, Dd and Ee. One haplotype consisting of c/C, d/D, e/E is inherited from each parent and the resulting Rhesus type of the individual depends on their inherited genotype. Now it is known that d does not exist and sometimes it is used in Fisher Race terminology to denote, the absence of D. The most common and important antigens are D, C, E, c, and e. D is the most immunogenic and in less than 3% of the individuals with D, C, E, c, and e antigens become immunogenic. Hence pre-transfusion testing for the other antigens is not routinely performed.

- In 1962, according to Rosenfield, the nomenclature is based on serological findings. As per Weiner, the Rh antigen product is from single gene.
- Persons whose red cells lack the D antigen, do not regularly have the corresponding antibody.
- Formation of **anti-D** antibodies almost always results from exposure of D-negative person by transfusion or pregnancy, to red cells with D antigen.
- The D antigen has greater immunogenicity. D negative persons, who receive a D positive transfusion, are expected to develop anti-D antibodies.

Genetics of Rh Blood Group

Despite its genetic complexity, the inheritance of the trait usually can be predicted by two alleles D. And the **Rh locus is on 1p36.11**. The Rh antigens are encoded by two genes RHD and RHCE. RHD encodes for D antigen, whereas RHCE encoded for Cc and Ee antigens. The d antigen does not exist and generally used to denote absence of D antigen. The genes (RHD and RHCE), both encode similar polypeptides of 417 amino acids with 12 membrane spanning domains.

Individuals who are **homozygous dominant (DD)** and **heterozygous (Dd)** are Rh positive. Those who are **homozygous recessive (dd)** are **Rh negative** (i.e they do not have the Rh antigen).

Serologic Testing for Rh Antigen

- To determine whether a person has genes that encoded D, C, c, E and e, the red cells are tested with antibody to each of the antigens.
- If the red cells express both C and c or both E and e, it can be assumed that the corresponding genes are present in the individual.
- If the red cells carry only C/c or only E/e the person is assumed to be homozygous for the particular allele.

Routine Rh typing for donors and patients involve only the D antigen.

Tests for the others Rh antigens are performed only for defined purpose such as:

a. Identifying unexpected Rh antibodies.
b. Obtaining compatible blood for a patient with an Rh antibody.
c. Investigating disputed parentage.
d. Isolating a panel of phenotypic cells for antibody identification.

Procedure

Now, monoclonal anti-D reagents have become widely available. Slide tests produce optimal results only when a high concentration of red cells and antibodies are combined at 37°C. (Refer to chapter on Blood Grouping).

Tube test for Rh testing

1. Place one drop of anti-D serum (polyclonal/monoclonal) in a clean test tube. (Refer to Fig. 4.6 ABO Blood Grouping and Rh typing by tube technique.)
2. Add one drop of 2–5% suspension of the red cells to be tested.
3. Mix gently and centrifuge for 30–45 sec at 1000 rpm.
4. Gently resuspend the cell button and examine for agglutination. Grade the reaction.

Interpretation

- Agglutination in anti-D tube indicates that the red cells in the tube are D-positive.
- If it has a smooth suspension, it is D-negative.

Matrix gel system for Rh typing: Anti-D (monoclonal IgM antibodies) gel card for testing Rh-D antigen are in use.

If Rh negative by above methods it has to be further tested for Du variant and if found negative it has to be labeled as Rh negative.

Weak or partial D

- **Weak D expression** primarily develops from **single point mutation of RhD gene**, reflected in the form of reduced number of D antigenic sites on the red cell membrane.

- **Red cells with partial D lack some antigenic sites** on extracellular portion of the RBC membrane.

Du: Weaker variant of D

- Du, the term was coined by Stratton in the year 1946.
- Donors/patient's with Du phenotype are Rh positive.
- Du antigen is less immunogenic than D antigen and can cause sensitization when given to D-negative individuals.
- With weak expression of D, most D positive red cells show clear cut macroscopic agglutination after centrifugation with reagent anti-D and can really be classified as D positive.
- For some D positive red cells, demonstration of the D antigen requires prolonged incubation with anti-D reagent or addition of anti-globulin serum after incubation with anti-D.
- These cells were classified as Du/weak D
- But use of monoclonal anti-D reagents have picked up many D positive compared to the older reagents.

Significance of weak D in blood transfusion

- Transfusion to D negative recipients with weak expression of the D antigen, such red cells could elicit an immune response to D.
- Du patients should receive Rh negative blood.

Du Test Procedure

Weak D expression can be recognized most reliably by anti-human globulin after incubation of the test red cells with anti-D. If the original test with anti-D was performed by tube testing, continue with the procedure.

1. **Mix and incubate** the tube for 15–30 min at 37°C in water bath.
2. Centrifuge for 15–60 sec × 1000 rpm.
3. Gently resuspend the cell bottom and examine them for agglutination.
4. If the test red cells are strongly agglutinated in the anti-D, record the sample as D positive.
5. If no agglutination, wash the cells for 3 times.

6. Add 1 drop of anti-IgG (AHG).

7. Mix centrifuge, view for agglutination under micro-scope.

Note: Du testing can also be performed with **Matrix gel system.**

Rh$_{null}$ phenotype: This is a rare variant of Rh system, when red cells do not express Rh antigens due to abnormal RHAG gene, which results in absence of Rh gene expression, RHD and RhC genes. These patients have red cell membrane abnormalities having stomatocytosis and haemolysis.

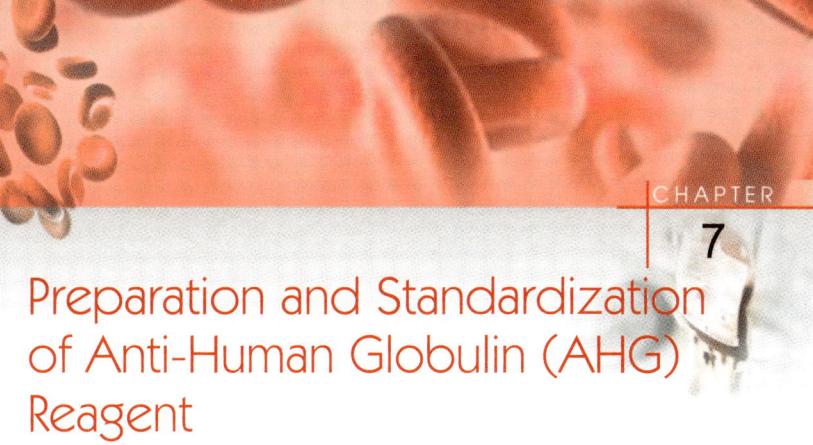

Preparation and Standardization of Anti-Human Globulin (AHG) Reagent

ANTI-HUMAN GLOBULIN REAGENT (*Coombs' Sera*)

- This is used to detect incomplete antibodies (IgG antibodies) which are capable of sensitising red cells but cannot agglutinate the same cells when suspended in saline as against to IgM antibodies.
- The technique can be used to detect the presence of antibodies or complement components that have been bound to the red cells *in vivo*, i.e. the **direct antiglobulin test (DAT, direct Coombs' test).**
- The test can detect IgG antibodies in the patient's serum. Incubate the serum with 'O' cells. The antibodies or complement will coat on these cells. Wash the cells and continue the procedure similar to DAT. This is **indirect antiglobulin test (IAT, indirect Coombs' test).**

PREPARATION OF AHG

Poly-specific AHG: Contains IgG and complement (C3b and C3d).

Anti-human globulin is prepared by injecting laboratory animals with human globulins or complements. Rabbits are the most suitable animals for immunization. Sheep and goats also can be used. This type of response produces polyclonal antibodies to IgG and complements. Polyclonal antibodies are mixture of antibodies produced from different clones of plasma cells. The resulting antibodies recognize different antigenic determinants (epitopes) week young rabbits with low titer of heteroagglutinins are ideal. Purified human IgG and C3 are injected. Alum precipitation method is commonly used. Animals are bled after 9–10 days after last injection. The antibodies produced are harvested.

Monospecific AHG: Contains only one antibody, may be anti-IgG, anti-C3d or anti-C3b.

The monoclonal antibodies are produced from hybridoma technology. Monoclonal antibodies are derived from one clone of plasma cells and can recognize only single epitope.

This is prepared by immunizing mice with purified human globulin or C3. After suitable immune response, the mouse splenic lymphocytes which are capable of secreting immuno-globulins are fused with myeloma cells. The hybridoma cells are screened for antibodies with required specificity and affinity.

Standardization of anti-human globulin reagent

- If IAT is undertaken with red cells suspended in normal ionic strength saline (NISS), maximum antibody is up-taken and hence maximum sensitivity is achieved in 60–90 minutes incubation period.
- The incubation period can be reduced to 10–15 minutes by using low ionic strength solutions (LISS). LISS–IAT is less sensitive than NISS
  - **IAT for identifying antibodies like anti-K** as the incubation period is reduced. **LISS–IAT if used in the cold, insignificant antibodies like anti-Pl, anti-Le** can be detected because of their increased **uptake at low ionic strength conditions**. Hence while using **LISS manufacturer's instructions** are followed strictly.
    LISS solution: This consists of 0.3 M glycine in 0.03 M sodium chloride. No buffer is added. The pH is 6.0.
- When IAT and DAT are performed in tubes, thorough washing (3 to 4 times) with large volume of saline is required before adding the antiglobulin reagent, as any free IgG or complement will neutralise the antiglobulin reagent.
- Prozone phenomena can give negative results and this can be eliminated by washing the cells after incubation with AHG or doing the test after diluting the serum.

- For the rare cases where the test is negative with poly-specific sera, it is necessary to test with monospecific sera having specific subclasses of anti-IgG, anti-C3b or anti-C3d. **Monospecific sera against IgM and subclasses of IgG** also can be prepared.
- In AHG anti-C4d should be avoided. So also, IgM antibodies should not be present. Each batch of reagents undergoes rigorous quality control at various stages of manufacture for its specificity, avidity and titre.

Poly-specific antiglobulin reagent containing **blend of anti-IgG, anti-C3b** and **anti-C3d** (anti-C3b and anti-C3d at controlled levels) are suitable for pre-transfusion testing, including crossmatch are recommended as per ISBT/ICSH guidelines.

Reagent storage and stability

a. Store the reagent at 2–8°C. DO NOT FREEZE.
b. The shelf life of the reagent is as per the expiry date mentioned on the reagent vial label.

The reagent contains sodium azide 0.1% as preservative. Avoid contact with skin and mucosa. On disposal, flush with large quantities of water.

Extreme turbidity may indicate microbial contamination or denaturation of protein due to thermal damage. Such reagents should be discarded.

Reagents are not from human source, hence contamination due to HBsAg and HIV is practically excluded.

Sample collection and storage

No special preparation of the patient is required prior to sample collection by approved techniques. **Do not use haemolysed samples.**

For direct antiglobulin test blood drawn into EDTA is preferred but oxalated or citrated blood also can be used. **The blood sample should be tested as soon as possible after collection and should not be stored. Stored blood can have C3d and Coombs' test can be positive.**

Coombs' Test

History

The antiglobulin test was first described in **1908 by Moreschi.** Introduced to human testing by **Coombs', Mourant and Race in 1945. Purpose**

- To detect IgG antibodies (incomplete antibodies) in the serum.
- To detect RBCs coated with antibodies.

Importance of Antiglobulin Test (Coombs' Test)

- Red cells coated with antibodies (IgG) will not agglutinate and these antibodies are too small to span the distance between the RBCs which are normally repelled by negative surface charges (zeta potential).
- Cells coated with only complement will not agglutinate.
- Anti-human globulin reagent solves this problem, when added to IgG/complement sensitized red cells the additional antibodies are able to bridge the gap between the red cells. Agglutination indicates presence of antibody/complement or both and information about strength of agglutination can be obtained. Grade the agglutination from 1+ to 4+, 4+ is the strong reaction.

Antiglobulin reagents

- Poly-specific Coombs' serum can recognise multiple epitopes on one antigen, and this contains anti-IgG and anti-C3 antibodies.

- Mono-specific Coombs' serum can detect only one epitope of antigen, specific against heavy chains of IgG, IgM and IgA or can detect only C3b or C3d.

Quality Control of Anti-globulin Reagents

ISBT/ICSH freeze dried reference reagent is used to evaluate the following:

- Specificity
- Potency of IgG
- Potency of anti-complement antibodies against C3b/ C3d present at controlled levels. No anti-C4d should be present.
- Free from false positive tests (stored blood cells uptake C3d, further augmented incubation with fresh serum).

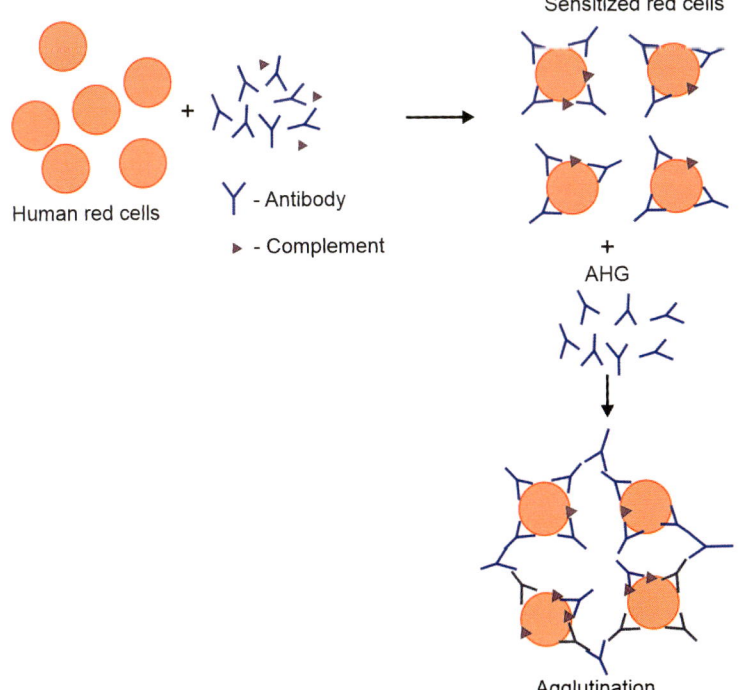

Human red cells +

Y - Antibody

▸ - Complement

Sensitized red cells

+
AHG

Agglutination

Fig. 8.1: Role of AHG in Coombs' test (direct antiglobulin test)

COOMBS' TEST

- Direct
- Indirect

Direct Test Performed Directly on the Red Cells

Indirect test name is a **misnomer**. In this test the patient's serum is tested for red cells antibodies.

Direct Coombs' Test/Direct Antiglobulin Test (DAT)

- This test is performed to detect anti-IgG antibody or other antibodies attached to the red cell surface within the blood stream.
- DAT is carried out in the following circumstances:
  - Transfusion reactions
  - Non-ABO antibodies
  - Drug-induced red cells sensitization
  - For example, pencillin, quinidine, α-methyldopa, cephalosporins
  - Autoimmune haemolytic anaemia
  - Paroxysmal cold haemoglobinuria (PCH) for presence of IgG/C3
  - Haemolytic disease of newborn

Precautions
- EDTA blood is preferred

Requirements
- Test tubes (10 × 75 mm)
- Pasteur pipettes
- Incubator
- Centrifuge
- AHG reagent
- Positive control cells (IgG coated)

Procedure
1. Prepare a 5% cell suspension in isotonic saline warmed at 37°C of the red blood cells to be tested. **Warm saline removes cold antibodies and non-specifically bound proteins**.

2. With clean pasture pipette add one drop of the prepared cell suspension to a small tube.
3. Wash three times with normal saline to remove all the traces of serum.
4. Decant completely after the last washing.
5. Add two drops of anti-human globulin serum.
6. Mix well and centrifuge for one minute at 1500 RPM.
7. Resuspend the cells by gentle agitation and examine macroscopically and microscopically for agglutination.
8. With negative reaction further incubated at room temperature, centrifuged and read again. This additional incubation promotes positive reaction with the presence of complement.
9. If negative, positive control cells (IgG coated) are added to the test tube. Agglutination confirms AHG is active.
10. Initial testing is done with poly-specific AHG and later can be confirmed with mono-specific AHG.

Indirect Coombs' Test (Indirect Antiglobulin Test)

This test is performed to detect the presence of Rh-antibodies or IgG antibodies produced in patients serum in case of the following:

To check whether an Rh-negative patient has developed
a. Rh-antibodies
b. Anti-Rh antibodies may be produced in the blood of any Rh-negative person by exposure to D antigen by:
    i. Transfusion of Rh positive blood
    ii. Pregnancy, if infant is Rh positive (when father is Rh-positive).
    iii. Abortion of Rh-positive fetus.
c. Rare blood groups which are similar to Rh blood group.

Rare blood groups which are similar to Rh blood group are mentioned below:
- MNSs—**anti-S and anti-sare IgG** class as a result of pregnancy or transfusion.
- Antibodies to **Lutheran antigens are IgG**.

- Antibodies to **Kell system antigens are IgG**
- **Duffy antibodies** are almost **exclusively IgG**
- Antibodies to the **Kidd antigens are almost exclusively IgG.**

Requirements
- Test tubes (10 × 75 mm)
- Pasteur pipettes
- Incubator
- Centrifuge

Specimen: Serum

Reagents
- Anti-human globulin serum
- Anti-D serum

Additional Requirements
- Coombs' control cells ('O' Rh (D) positive cells).
- Make a pooled 'O' Rh (D) positive cells from at least three different 'O' positive blood samples.
- Wash these cells three times in normal saline (these cells should be completely free from serum with no free anti-bodies). Make 5% saline suspension of these cells.

Procedure
1. Label three test tubes as 'T'' (test serum), PC (positive control) and NC (negative control).
2. In the tube labeled as 'T', add two drops of serum
3. In the tube 'NC', add one drop of saline
4. In the tube PC, add positive serum.
5. Add one drop of 5 % saline suspension of the pooled 'O' Rh (D) positive cells in each tube.
6. Incubate all the three tubes for one hour at 37°C.
7. Wash the cells three times in normal saline to remove excess serum with no free antibodies, (in the case of inadequate washings of the red cells, negative results may be obtained).
8. Add two drops of Coombs' serum (anti-human serum) to each tube. Keep for 5 minutes and then centrifuge at 1,500 RPM for one minute.

9. Re-suspend the cells and examine macroscopically as well as microscopically.

Test interpretation

Test	Observations	Conclusions
Positive Control (PC)	Agglutination	Correctly performed test procedure.
	No agglutination	Coombs' serum may not be proper, repeat the test again
Negative Control (NC)	It should show no agglutination, since saline does not contain anti-D or any other antibodies.	
Test serum (T)	Agglutination	Patient's serum contains anti-D
	If PC results are correct, no agglutination	Patient's serum does not contain anti-D

- Poly-specific AHG sera can detect
  - Anti-IgG, anti-C3 antibodies
- Mono-specific AHG can detect only IgG/ IgM / IgA/C3

False positive test
- Clotted blood at cold temp. or room temp.
- Hospitalized patients can have anti-C3d
- If clotted sample, complement can bound to the red cells and test can give positive test.

False negative test
- Failure to wash the red cells properly, AHG neutralized by the immunoglobulins or complement.
- Excessive agitation may breakup agglutinates at reading stage.
- Use of impotent antisera, such that weakly sensitised cells not detected.
- Use of antisera lacking the antibody corresponding to the subclass of immunoglobulin responsible for sensitisation.
- Not adding AHG.
- Improper centrifugation.
- Improper storage, bacterial contamination, and contamination with human serum will impair AHG reagent activity.

- Presence of an antibody which can be readily eluted during washing.

New technology for detection of antibodies by antiglobulin test

1. Solid phase red cell adherence method: Sensitized red cells are immobilized on solid matrix.
2. Column agglutination technique (matrix gel method): Microtubes contain dextran acrylamide gel particles or Gel bead and AHG to which the donor cells are added. After centrifugation; agglutinated red cells are trapped at the top. Non-agglutinated red cells will be at the bottom.

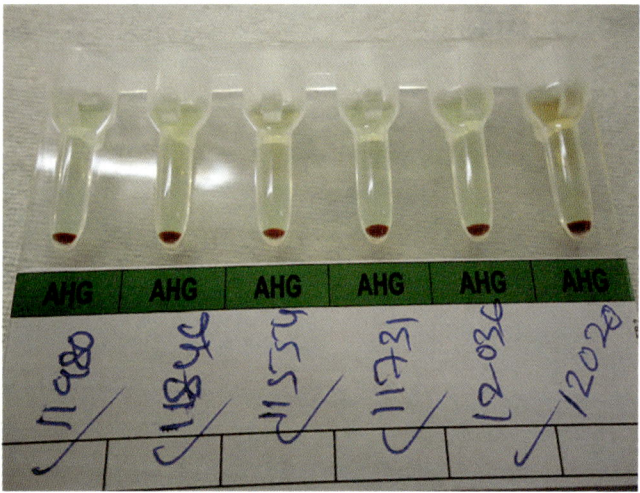

Fig. 8.2: Coombs' test matrix gel method

Thus, Coombs' test detects incomplete antibodies (IgG) and C3 or both in the serum or on the red cell surface.

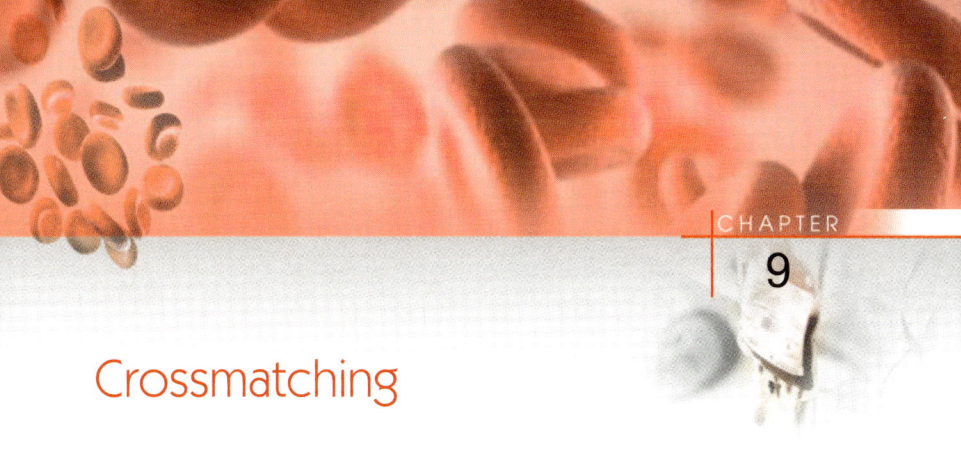

Crossmatching

AIM OF CROSSMATCHING

The procedure is used to determine compatibility between donor and recipients' blood, i.e. to check for haemolysis or any agglutination if they are mixed together. With accurate blood grouping, Rh typing of recipient and selection of donor with same blood groups, the two bloods are to be compatible.

However, there are occasions when,

- The recipient may have antibodies in his serum.
- The donor may have antibodies in his serum.
- There may be mistake in performing, reading and recording of blood groups and Rh typing.

Major Crossmatch

Donor's red cells are mixed with recipient's serum. This procedure determines compatibility between red cells of donor and serum (plasma) of the recipient.

Minor Crossmatch

Donor's serum is mixed with recipient's red cells. This procedure determines compatibility between serum (plasma) of donor and red cells of the recipient. However, this is not used routinely.

Immediate spin crossmatch may be preferred when:

1. No clinically significant unexpected antibodies are detected in the antibody screen.

2. No record of previous detection of clinically significant unexpected antibodies.

This procedure requires patient's serum to be mixed with saline suspended red cells (2–4% conc.) of donor at room temperature. The centrifuge immediately (1000 rpm for 1 minute or 3400 rpm for 20 seconds).

If clinically significant antibodies are present, the crossmatch technique should include incubation at 37°C followed by the anti-globulin test.

Procedure

1. Prepare 5% cell suspension of patients and donor cells in two separate test tubes.
2. **Major crossmatch:** In a test tube, add two drops of patient's serum and one drop of donor cells.
3. **Minor crossmatch:** In a test tube add two drops of donor serum and one drop of patient's cells.
4. Mix the contents; keep the tubes at room temp. for 30 minutes. Centrifuge at 1500 rpm × 1 minute.
5. If no agglutination, then it is compatible.

Major crossmatch by matrix gel system:

1. Identify the card with recipient's/donor's name or number.
2. Take out the aluminium foil.
3. Add **50 μl donor cell suspension** (0.8%) to the microtube.
4. Add 25 μl of recipient's plasma/serum.
5. Incubate at 37°C × 15 minutes.
6. Centrifuge at 1200 rpm for 10 min.
7. Read the reaction.

Indirect Anti-globulin Test for Major Crossmatch

In the first step of anti-globulin crossmatch is similar to imme-diate spin crossmatch. Addition of albumin acts as potentiator.

Procedure

Initial phase

1. Label two test tubes as A (for albumin) and B (for saline), depending upon the number of donors to be crossmatched, as many pairs of such labeled tubes would be required.

2. Prepare a 5% suspension of the red cells to be tested in isotonic saline.

3. Pipette two drops of recipient serum in both the labeled test tubes.

4. Pipette one drop of donor red cells in both the labeled test tubes and mix well.

5. Only to the albumin tube (A) add two drops of bovine albumin reagent and mix well.

6. Centrifuge both the tubes for one minute at 1000 rpm or for 20 seconds at 3400 rpm.

7. Observe for haemolysis. Re-suspend the cell button and observe for agglutination macroscopically.

8. Proceed to incubation phase.

9. Prepare a 5% suspension of the red cells to be tested in isotonic saline.

10. Pipette two drops of recipient serum in both the labeled test tubes.

11. Only to the albumin tube (A) add two drops of bovine albumin reagent and mix well.

12. Centrifuge both the tubes for one minute at 1000 rpm or for 20 seconds at 3400 rpm.

13. Observe for haemolysis. Re-suspend the cell button and observe for agglutination macroscopically.

14. Proceed to incubation phase.

Incubation phase

1. Incubate the saline tube at room temperature and the albumin tube at 37°C for fifteen minutes (up to 30 minutes).

2. Re-suspend the cell button and observe for agglutination macroscopically.

3. Proceed to anti-globulin phase.

Anti-globulin phase

1. Only the albumin tubes (A) are tested in the anti-globulin phase.

2. Wash the mixture of red blood cells and serum thoroughly with isotonic saline for minimum of three times. Decant completely after the last wash.

3. Place two drops of anti-human globulin reagent into the test tubes containing the sedimented cells and mix well.

4. Centrifuge for one minute at 1000 rpm or 20 seconds at 3400 rpm. Very gently, re-suspend the cell button and observe for agglutination macroscopically.

COOMBS' TEST IN ANTIBODY IDENTIFICATION

Direct Anti-globulin Test

Agglutination of red blood cells is a positive test result and indicates presence of IgG antibodies or components of complement on the red blood cells.

No agglutination is a negative test result and indicates absence of IgG antibodies or components of complement on the red blood cells.

Indirect Anti-globulin Test

In all phases of the compatibility test, if no agglutination or haemolysis is observed, then the patient and the donor may be considered compatible. If haemolysis or agglutination at any point till the completion of the anti-globulin phase is observed, the patient and the donor are considered incompatible.

Note:

1. If plasma is used in the indirect anti-globulin test, the complement dependent antibodies may not be detected due to the absence of calcium.

2. To all negative test results, after the antiglobulin test phase, one drop of Coombs' control cells should be added. If Coombs' control cells do not agglutinate, then the compatibility test must be repeated.

3. In the indirect antiglobulin test procedure, an auto-control tube (individual's cells in his own serum) should run.

4. Red blood cells showing a positive direct anti-globulin test cannot be used for the indirect anti-globulin test.

5. It is recommended that anti-IgG activity of the anti-human globulin reagent be tested from time to time preferably on a daily basis using Coombs' control cells as a positive control.

6. All glassware used in the test should be scrupulously clean, dry and free from contamination with human serum.

7. Contaminated bovine serum albumin, saline or glassware may inactivate anti-human globulin reagent.

8. Use of various drugs and certain diseases (such as megaloblastic anaemia) are known to be associated with a positive direct anti-globulin test.

9. Cord cells obtained from a newborn exhibiting haemolytic disease of the newborn, especially due to ABO incompatibility may give false negative results.

10. Anti-human globulin reagent should not contain anti-C4 and is free from anti-T activity.

11. As under centrifugation or over centrifugation could lead to erroneous results, it is recommended that each laboratory calibrate its own equipment and the time required for achieving the desired results.

Note: Addition of albumin (22%, 30%, polymerized bovine serum) prior to incubation at 37°C has been used to enhance the sensitivity of antibody detection tests. In particular, direct agglutination by Rh antibodies after incubation at 37°C appears to be enhanced.

Transfusion Reactions

Definition

A transfusion reaction is defined as any unfavorable event that occurs during or after a transfusion of blood and its components.

Classification of Transfusion Reactions

Transfusion reactions can be classified as follows:
1. Acute and delayed: These are again subdivided into immunological and non-immunological
2. Depending upon the severity as:
   a. Mild reactions
   b. Moderately severe reactions, and
   c. Life-threatening reactions

ACUTE TRANSFUSION REACTIONS—IMMUNOLOGICAL

- Febrile non-haemolytic transfusion reaction (FNHTR)
- Allergic reactions
- Anaphylactic and anaphylactoid reactions
- Acute haemolytic transfusion reactions (AHTRs)
- Transfusion related acute lung injury (TRALI)

ACUTE TRANSFUSION REACTIONS—NON-IMMUNOLOGICAL

- Bacterial contamination
- Transfusion-associated circulatory overload (TACO)
- Physical and chemical haemolysis
- Metabolic derangements

Delayed Transfusion Reactions—Immunological

- Delayed haemolytic transfusion reactions (DHTRs)
- Transfusion-associated graft-versus-host disease (TA-GvHD)
- Post-transfusion purpura

Delayed Transfusion Reactions—Non-immunological

- Iron overload
- Post-transfusion haemosiderosis
- Transfusion-transmitted diseases

Common Signs and Symptoms

Common signs	Symptoms
Nausea	Heat at infusion site
Chills	Itching
Coughing	Myalgia
Cyanosis	Hypotension
Dyspnea	Oliguria/anuria
Facial flushing	Pulmonary edema
Fever (>1°C)	Wheezing
Headache	Chest/back pain
Urticaria	Abnormal bleeding
Rash	Hemoglobinuria
Uneasy feeling	

FEBRILE NON-HAEMOLYTIC TRANSFUSION REACTION (FNHTR)

This is a frequent kind of reaction, occurs in 1:200 cases.

Definition

There is increase of 1°C temperature or more associated with transfusion of blood when there is no medical explanation for fever other than blood transfusion.

Causes

Patient has immunologic sensitization to donor WBCs, platelets or plasma proteins.

Common Sources

Prior transfusions, previous pregnancies, previous transplants.

Pathophysiology

This is caused from **HLA class I antigens or leucocyte antigens on the WBCs of the donor** that react with the recipient's antibodies (blood components with WBCs) and activate complement system which releases cytokines (IL-1, IL-6, and TNF). These act on thermoregulatory center in hypothalamus and responsible for increase in temperature.

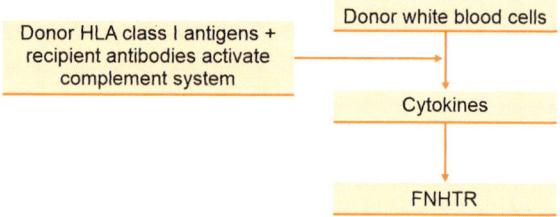

Signs and Symptoms

- Fever with or without chills, with increase of 1 degree C to 2 degree C temperature.
- Most symptoms are mild.
- With severe reaction there can be hypotension, cyanosis, tachycardia, tachypnea, dyspnea, cough, etc.
- There can be headache, flushing, anxiety, muscle pain.

Prevention

- Anti-pyretics are used to treat fever or are given prior to blood transfusion as a preventive measure.
- Discontinue blood transfusion if the patient has severe reaction.
- Pre-storage leucocyte reduced units of red blood cell or platelet packs may also be given. Leucocyte reduced units should have the following:
    a. As per the standards, minimum of 85 percent red cell recovery should be ensured in 95 units tested.
    b. The whole blood unit should have less than 5×10^6 white blood cells. This is log 3 reduction.
    c. This is best achieved by 3rd and 4th generation filters.

Note: Also refer to topic on "safe use of blood".

ALLERGIC REACTIONS

This is a frequent kind of reaction.

Causes

Exact mechanism for sensitization is not known.

Patient is sensitized (usually IgE antibody) to foreign plasma antigens. Commonly caused by transfusion of plasma containing blood components, e.g. FFP, cryoprecipitate, platelet concentrates.

Pathophysiology

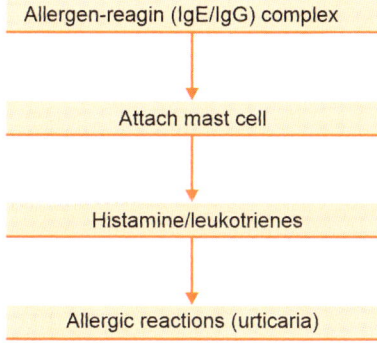

Signs and Symptoms

- Flushing
- Headache
- Itching
- Urticaria
- Rarely, angioedema—epiglottal oedema; bronchial airway constriction, hypotension, dyspnea and rales.
  This is not life threatening.

Management

Pre-medicate patient with anti-histamines.

If signs/symptoms are mild and/or transient, restart transfusion after treatment.

Do **NOT** restart transfusion if pulmonary symptoms/signs and fever are present.

Prevention

- Use plasma deficient blood components.
- Prophylactically treat with antihistamines.

Note: Also refer to topic on "Safe use of blood".

ANAPHYLACTIC AND ANAPHYLACTOID REACTIONS

Anaphylaxis can range from mild urticaria to severe shock and death although rare. These occur at the rate of about 1 per 150,000 patients.

Pathophysiology

Pre-formed anti-IgA antibodies are present in the recipient's blood with IgA deficiency which reacts with IgA present in the donor plasma.

Signs and Symptoms

Anaphylactic reactions: Coughing, dyspnea, nausea, emesis, bronchospasm, flushing of skin, hypotension, abdominal cramps, diarrhoea, cardiac arrest, shock, and death.

Anaphylactoid reactions (less severe): Urticaria, periorbital swelling, dyspnea, or peri-laryngeal oedema.

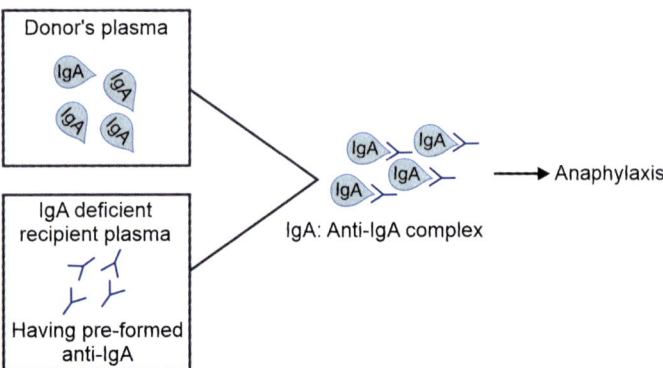

Fig. 10.1: Anaphylaxis in IgA deficient recipient with pre-formed IgA antibodies, when transfused with donor having IgA

Therapy and Prevention

- Stop transfusion.
- Keep IV line open.
- Medication: Use epinephrine (vasoconstrictors and broncho-dilators) and corticosteroids.
- Use washed RBCs and blood components.
- Transfuse IgA deficient blood.

ACUTE HAEMOLYTIC TRANSFUSION REACTIONS (AHTRs)

Most common cause for AHTR is ABO incompatibility often due to clerical error.

Incidence: 1:25,000.

As little as 10–15 mL can trigger a reaction. Occurs within 24 hours.

Causes

- Transfusion **of incompatible donor RBCs into patient**.
- Usually an ABO incompatibility, most commonly **antibodies of A, B or AB**.
- Red cell destruction due to **complement activation by IgM antibodies**. Antibodies in patient plasma attach to antigens on donor RBCs causing RBC destruction intra-vascularly.
- Potent anaphylatoxins including **C3a and C5a are released, later form membrane attack factor.**
- C3a and C5a cause hypotension.
- Mast cells release **histamine and serotonin which constricts small arteries and arterioles** leading to **renal ischemia.**
- **Release** of bradykinin causes vasodilatation and increased vascular permeability.
- Release of **cytokines like TNF-α, IL-1 and IL-8 induces hypotension.**
- Antigen and antibody interaction has effects on **coagulation cascade** causing disseminated intravascular coagulation (DIC).

Signs and Symptoms of AHTR

Signs	Symptoms
Chills	Fever
Facial flushing	Dyspnea
Hypotension	Generalized bleeding
Renal failure	Haemoglobinemia
DIC	Haemoglobinuria
Shock	Nausea
Chest pain	Vomiting
Pain along infusion vein	Back pain

Differential Diagnosis for AHTR

- Microbial contamination
- Physical/chemical/drug related damage to stored RBCs
- Auto-immune haemolytic anaemia

Steps to be taken when a transfusion reaction occurs due to AHTR:

- Stop the transfusion immediately.
- An intravenous line with normal saline should be maintained.
- Obtain vital signs.
- Begin O_2 if pulmonary symptoms are prominent.
- Obtain a new blood sample for repeat ABO compatibility test and for evidence of haemolysis.
- Obtain a urine sample, if the patient can void.
- Obtain a chest X-ray if pulmonary symptoms are prominent.
- Physician is notified.
- Bedside clerical checks of all forms, labels and patient identification for correctness of the unit and the intended recipient are required.
- The unit and all tubing should be returned to the blood bank, along with post-infusion blood and urine samples.
- Finally, the reaction should be documented in the patient's chart.
- Once these initial measures have been implemented, the investigation of the reaction by the transfusion service can proceed.

This type of reaction is a most dangerous immunologic complication of red cell unit transfusion.

- It carries high risk of morbidity or mortality.
- Morbidity is because of renal failure and DIC.
- Mortality: Occurs in 1 per 100,000 transfusions.

Management

- Treat hypotension, renal failure, DIC, etc.
- Submit blood samples for blood bank/laboratory tests.
- Avoid, if possible, further transfusions till work-up is complete and/or patient recovers from reaction.
- To prevent renal failure, fluids (saline) are infused along with diuretics to increase urine output.

Prevention

Preventing or detecting errors in every phase of the transfusion process such as:
- Sample acquisition
- At all steps in laboratory testing
- At the time of issue
- At the time of transfusion
- Good manufacturing practices with written standard operating procedures should be followed.
- Perform pre-transfusion compatibility testing.
- Ensure that all clinical staff to recognize signs and symptoms of acute haemolytic transfusion reaction.

Laboratory Investigations in AHTRs

On pre-transfusion sample: Re-confirm ABO, Rh and antibody screen tests.

On post-transfusion sample: Following are to be undertaken.
- ABO, Rh, antibody screen
- DCT
- Urine for haemoglobinuria
- Serum bilirubin
- Haemoglobinaemia (>50 mg/dL)

- Blood urea, creatinine
- Urine output
- Coagulation screen
- Identify discrepancies

Note: Also refer to topic on "Safe use of blood".

TRANSFUSION RELATED ACUTE LUNG INJURY (TRALI)

This occurs in 1 in 5,000 transfusions.

Symptoms occur within 2 hours and may end in 2–4 days if treated.

Patient displays **acute respiratory insufficiency** with X-ray showing bilateral symmetric **pulmonary oedema.**

Pathophysiology

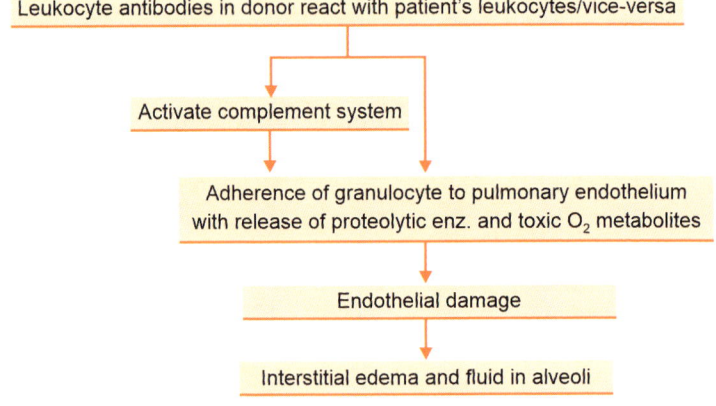

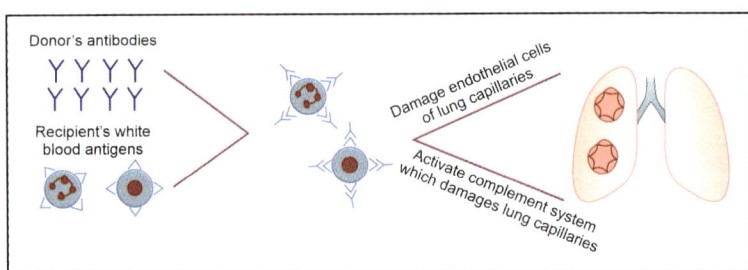

Fig. 10.2: Pathophysiology of TRALI with damage to endothelial cells in lung.

Donor antibodies activate recipient's WBCs or vice versa which cause damage to blood vessels in lung tissue.

Then fluids and proteins leak into alveolar space/interstitium. Mechanism is similar to ARDS.

Non-cardiogenic bilateral pulmonary oedema develops.

Signs and Symptoms

- Severe dyspnea, cyanosis, tachycardia, and hypoxemia
- Hypotension
- Fever
- Chills

Prevention

- Avoid donations from multiparous women and those who have received multiple transfusions.
- Transfuse washed RBCs from which plasma is removed.
- Platelet units can also be washed, but platelet function is significantly reduced.

Management

- Steroids: Treat with IV steroids, although they may not work well.
- Aggressive ventilatory support.
- Haemodynamic support.

Note: Also refer to topic on "safe use of blood".

BACTERIAL CONTAMINATION

- Does not involve antigen–antibody interactions.
- Results from bacterial contamination of blood and blood products.

Red cells can be contaminated by:

1. Gram-negative rods (those produce endotoxins and grow in cold temperature), following are most common.
   - *Yersinia enterocolitica*
   - *Serratia liquefaciens, E. coli*
   - *Serratia*
   - *Pseudomonas*

2. Gram-positive cocci (less common)
   - *Staphylococcus epidermidis*
   - *Staphylococcus aureus*

Platelets can be contaminated by

Majority are Gram-negative cocci,
- Gram-negative rods can also contaminate.
- Organisms listed above are also included.

Plasma products
- Uncommonly contaminated
- Rarely pseudomonas may contaminate

Pathophysiology

Bacteria growing in cold and room temperature produce toxins.

Symptoms and Signs

- Acute onset within 30 minutes after transfusion.
- Dryness and flushing of skin.
- Fever, hypotension, shaking chills, muscle pain, vomiting, abdominal cramps, bloody diarrhoea, haemoglobinuria, shock, renal failure, and DIC.

Management

- Stop transfusion immediately and treat with antibiotics.
- Hypotension can be treated with vasopressors and treat accordingly depending on severity.

Therapy

- Stop transfusion
- Broad spectrum antibiotics
- Treat hypotension
- Symptomatic treatment
- Prevention: Care during phlebotomy and blood components preparation and processing, thawing by sterile technique should be undertaken.

Note: Also refer to topic on "Safe use of blood".

TRANSFUSION ASSOCIATED CIRCULATORY OVERLOAD (TACO)

Patients at significant risk are:

- Children
- Elderly patients
- Chronic anaemia
- Cardiac disease
- Thalassemia major, sickle cell disease or congenital haemolytic anaemias

Pathophysiology

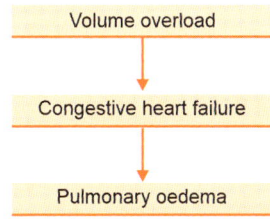

Symptoms and Signs

Symptoms	Signs
Dyspnea	Chest discomfort
Coughing	Headache
Cyanosis	Restlessness
Orthopnea	Tachycardia
Systolic hypertension	

Therapy

- Rapid reduction of hypervolemia
- Respiratory and cardiac support
- Oxygen therapy
- Diuretics
- Therapeutic phlebotomy

Prevention

- Use appropriate transfusion rate. Run slowly, small aliquots in 4 hr and subsequently within 24 hr.
- Use appropriate blood components.

Note: Also refer to topic on "Safe use of blood".

PHYSICAL AND CHEMICAL HAEMOLYSIS

Following are the causes:

Improper storage: Overheating or freezing.

Improper preparation: Freezing without cryoprotective agent.

Mechanical stress: Cardio-pulmonary bypass pump.

Simultaneous mixing of blood with drugs/hypotonic (5% dextrose)/hypertonic solutions (50% dextrose).

METABOLIC DERANGEMENTS

- Citrate toxicity
- Hyperkalemia
- Hypothermia
- Coagulopathy in massive transfusion
- Air embolism

Note:

- These have synergistic effects.
- Blood warmer can prevent hypothermia.
- Slow infusion rate is required.

DELAYED HAEMOLYTIC TRANSFUSION REACTIONS (DHTRs)

- DHTRs may not be recognised for weeks or months after transfusion. This is due to anamnestic reaction mediated by IgG antibodies on the following occasions.
    - Patient previously exposed to RBC antigen and has low antibody titer until exposed again.
    - Antibodies to Rh, Kidd, Duffy, and Kell blood groups.
- DAT is negative at first, but becomes positive later.
- Tests are performed to identify antibody.
- Patient may be asymptomatic.
- Fever and anaemia 2–14 days after transfusion are due to DHTRs.

Symptoms

- Fever
- Mild jaundice

Investigations

- Reduced haemoglobin more rapid than usual
- Falling Hct/PCV
- Reticulocytosis
- Haemoglobinuria
- High bilirubin
- Positive DAT in 50% of the cases
  These patients must be given antigen negative blood.

Differential Diagnosis

- TA-GvHD
- Transfusion-induced malaria

Prevention

- Check the previous records for alloimmunization.
- Antigen negative blood to be transfused.

TRANSFUSION-ASSOCIATED GRAFT-VERSUS-HOST DISEASE (TA-GvHD)

Patients at risk are:

- Immuno-compromised patients
- Newborn and geriatric patients
- Patients with bone marrow transplantation
- Patients on chemotherapy
- Patients with radiation treatment
- Patients who receive relatives' blood

Pathophysiology

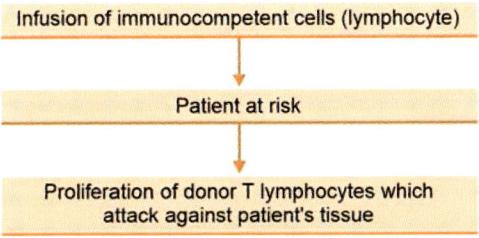

Signs and Symptoms

- Onset—3 to 30 days after transfusion.
- Clinically significant pancytopenia.
- Other effects include fever, rise in liver enzyme, copious watery diarrhoea, erythematous skin, erythroderma and desquamation.

Therapy

Drugs: Corticosteroids, methotrexate, azathioprine, antithymocyte globulin.

Prevention

- No adequate therapy available.
- Irradiation of blood components is safer.
- Avoid potential fatalities.
- Avoid relatives' blood
- Rare but fatal condition that has 90% mortality rate.
- Symptoms appear usually after about 12 days.
- Caused by donor lymphocytes, which are transfused into an immune-compromised recipient.
- **Pancytopenia** occurs as a result of the immunologic response.
- Any components that contain T-lymphocytes should be irradiated to prevent GVHD.

POST-TRANSFUSION PURPURA

- Rare complication
- Rapid onset of thrombocytopenia as a result of anamnestic production of platelet alloantibody.
- Usually occurs in multiparous women who do not have the antigen.

Pathophysiology

Platelet antibody (anti-PLA1), attaches on platelet surface and causes destruction of platelets by reticuloendothelial system.

Signs and Symptoms

- Purpura and thrombocytopenia occur.
- Occur 1–2 weeks after transfusion.
- The platelet count drops to <10,000 cells/cmm

Therapy and Prevention

- Corticosteroids
- Exchange transfusion
- Plasmapheresis
- Cerebral haemorrhage is a major concern

IRON OVERLOAD AND HAEMOSIDEROSIS

- 1 unit of packed red cells has 250 mg of iron.
- Iron that can be removed by the body—1 mg/day.
- Thus, with multiple transfusions iron accumulates in tissues and causes haemosiderosis.
- Post-transfusion haemosiderosis—affected organs: Heart, liver, endocrine glands.

Signs and Symptoms

Muscle weakness, fatigue, weight loss, mild jaundice, anaemia, mild diabetes, and cardiac arrhythmia

- Occurs in individuals who receive multiple transfusions.
- Excess iron accumulates in macrophages in various tissues (liver, heart, endocrine glands).
- It appears as dark brown granules in the cells.
- May lead to organ failure.
- Therapy: Iron-chelating agents.
- Prevention: Transfuse with young RBCs.

TRANSFUSION TRANSMITTED DISEASES (TTDs)

Blood transfusion can transmit diseases and the list of possible transmitted diseases is given below:

Viral Infections

Hepatitis viruses: HBV, HCV

Retroviruses: HIV

Herpes viruses: CMV, EBV

Parvovirus: Human B19 parvovirus

Prion: Infectious particle of CJD

Other viruses: West Nile disease

Bacterial Infection

Gram-negative and Gram-positive bacteria.

Syphilis

- Lyme disease (Borrelliosis)
- Parasitic infections
  - Malaria
  - Chagas' disease
  - Toxoplasmosis
  - Leishmaniasis

Note: For details refer to chapter on **transfusion transmitted diseases (TTDs).**

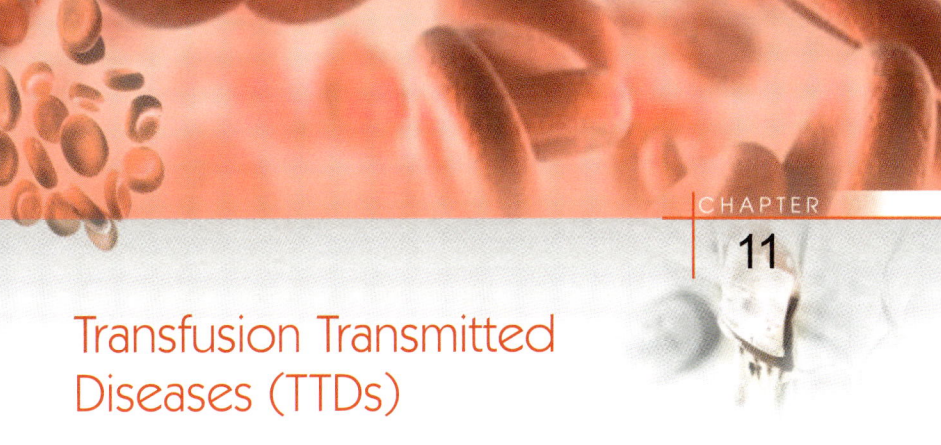

Transfusion Transmitted Diseases (TTDs)

TRANSFUSION TRANSMITTED DISEASES/INFECTIONS (TTDs/TTIs)

With increasing knowledge about mode of spread amongst population, the HIV infection has reduced. However, In the year 2015, India is estimated to have around 86000 new HIV cases, showing 66% decline in new infections compared to the year 2000 and 32% decline from 2007; the total number of people living with HIV in India is estimated to be 21.17 lakhs.[4]

As per the rules of Indian Government and National Aids Prevention and Control policy, testing of every unit of blood is mandatory and the blood collected is screened using highest quality screening tests for 5 TTIs/TTDs, namely:

- HIV 1 and 2
- Hepatitis C virus (HCV)
- Hepatitis B virus (HBV)
- Malaria
- Syphilis

FDA in USA requires infectious disease tests to be tested for HIV 1 and 2, HBV, HCV, human T cell lymphoma leukemia (HTLV) I and II, syphilis and West Nile Virus (WNV) and nucleic acid testing (NAT) for HIV, HBV, HCV and WNV (as per AABB standards).

Due to prevalence of AIDS virus, the Ministry of Health and Family Welfare (Government of India) issued a notification in the year 1989 under the Drugs and Cosmetics Rules and made the test HIV 1 and 2 antibodies of whole human blood as mandatory requirement before transfusion.

In the year 1990, blood and blood products were regulated by the Government of India and 3 laboratories, viz. NICD Delhi, NIV Pune and CMC Vellore, were notified to function as laboratories under 3A of Drugs and Cosmetics Rules to test HIV antibodies.

As trained technicians were not available in the blood banks to carry out the test for HIV 1 and 2 antibodies, the Ministry of Health and Family Welfare notified 112 Surveillance Centers to act as testing laboratories for the blood banks for carrying out the above tests.

Questionnaire for donors is provided and this is:
- To find out if the donor is having any transmissible diseases.
- TTDs/TTIs are deferrals; some are permanent and some temporary.
- The aim of blood transfusion is to do good to the patient.
- Thus, screening of blood for infectious diseases is essential.

Signs and symptoms of AIDS and high risk activities, foreign travel, recent vaccination, drug history, window periods of infections, etc. are to be looked for.

Donors must document accurate information. The donors should understand the donation process, blood testing and that the blood donation is a voluntary informed decision.

Do not donate blood to be tested for a HIV/AIDS, hepatitis or any other infectious disease.

Counseling for "reactive" donors: If a blood sample tests positive for any TTI, then
- Tests are repeated in duplicate.
- Complete confidentiality is maintained about the test results.
- Only the donor is informed, counselled and encouraged for further testing.

Confidentiality/Counselling

The data will be kept confidential, except where required by law. If the blood tests are positive to any of the administered standard tests, patient will receive confidential notification. The blood bank maintains strict confidentiality of all blood donor records.

MALARIA

Malaria is one of the major public health problems of the country. Around 1.5 million confirmed cases are reported annually by the National Vector Borne Disease Control Programme (NVBDCP), of which 40–50% are due to *Plasmodium falciparum*.[5]

Malaria is transmitted easily through infected RBCs. Many donors are unaware that they have malaria, which may be latent and is transmissible by blood donation.

Prospective donors must be asked about malaria or whether they had been to a region (endemic area) where it is prevalent.

Donors who have had a diagnosis of malaria or who are immigrants, refugees, or citizens from countries in which malaria is considered endemic are deferred for 3 years; travelers to endemic countries are deferred for 1 year.

Malaria is curable if effective treatment is started early. Delay in treatment may lead to serious consequences including death.

Prompt and effective treatment is also important for controlling the transmission of malaria.

A revised National Drug Policy on malaria has been adopted by the Ministry of Health and Family Welfare in 2008 and these guidelines have therefore been prepared for clinicians to treat malaria.

Microscopy of stained thick and thin blood smears remains the gold standard for confirmation of diagnosis of malaria.

The advantages of microscopy are:

The sensitivity is high. It is possible to detect malarial parasites at low densities. It also helps to quantify the parasite load.

It is possible to distinguish the various species of malaria parasite and their different stages.

Malaria: Rapid Diagnostic Tests (RDT)

Rapid diagnostic tests are based on the detection of circulating parasite antigens. Several types of RDTs are available. Some of them can only detect *P. falciparum*, while others can detect *P. vivax* and other species as well.

RDTs are produced by different companies, so there may be differences in the contents and in the manner in which the test is done.

The user's manual should always be read properly and instructions followed meticulously. The results should be read at specified time. The kits should be within expiry date and should be transported and stored under recommended conditions.

Histidine-rich protein 2 (HRP2-*P. falciparum*), and p-lactate dehydrogenase (pLDH-*P. vivax*) are usually tested.

The kits are expensive and temperature sensitive. Presently, NVBDCP supplies RDT kits for detection of *P. falciparum* at locations where microscopy results are not obtainable within 24 hours of sample collection.

Failure to observe these criteria can lead to false negative results. It should be noted that Pf HRP2-based kits may show positive result up to three weeks of successful treatment.

ELISA for Malaria

ELISA detects malaria genus specific pLDH released by parasitized blood cells.

The microwells are coated with monoclonal anti-pLDH antibodies. Another anti-pLDH antibody is biotinylated.

Samples along with positive and negative controls are added in the microwells and incubated with biotinylated antibody.

The wells are washed to remove unbound components.

Procedure of ELISA

100 μl sample diluent containing antibody.

25 μl control/whole blood.

Shake gently.

Incubate for 30 min at 37°C. Wash with buffer.

Add 100 μl diluted conjugate. Incubate for 30 min at room temperature.

Wash 6 times.

100 μl of substrate and incubate for 30 min at room temperature.

100 μl of stop solution.

Read the absorbance at 450 nm with 600–700 nm as reference within 30 min after stop solution.

Positive or negative reading is given according to the cut-off value which is calculated as per the manufacture's manual.

PCR using a modification of the technique originally described by Snounou et. al. with primers targeting the *Plasmodium* spp. 18S rRNA genes can be used.[6]

Nested PCR is more sensitive compared to microscopy, allowing the detection of *Plasmodium* in cases with low parasitemia, as well as mixed infections of malaria. In all instances, specimens that are PCR positive and microscopy negative depict symptomatic patients with a history of travel to malaria areas of endemicity.

Nested PCR can detect mixed infection with *P. falciparum* and *P. ovale* that was missed by microscopy.

The nested PCR can detect all four species of *Plasmodium*. Nested PCR is valuable as a confirmatory test and implementation should be considered by reference laboratories and worldwide with adequate laboratory infrastructure to perform molecular procedures.

Molecular techniques are costly procedures, including the cost of labor and reagents, compared to the examination of blood smears. This represents a true impairment for its implementation in reference laboratories located in poor regions of the world where malaria is endemic.

HIV INFECTION

HIV infection was recognized only in 1981. AIDS has rapidly established itself throughout the world.

In the year 2001, number of adults/children living with AIDS worldwide was 40 millions. In 2012, it was 35.3 millions. Dying with AIDS worldwide was 3 millions in 2001 and in 2012 it was 1.6 millions.[7]

- In developed nations, number is decreasing due to combined anti-retroviral therapy.
- In India, infection is seen in the 2nd to 3rd decade with increasing number of males being affected with subsequent infection to wife and children.

- **Blood is** the source of infection for HIV/AIDS. Risk of HIV from contaminated blood transfusion is 95%. Contaminated blood, transfusion of whole blood, platelets, factors VIII and IX (derived from plasma) are the sources for HIV/AIDS.
- Drug addicts have high risk of HIV due to sharing of needles.
- Skin piercing (including injections, ear piercing, tattooing, acupuncture) are at high risk to this disease.

Laboratory Diagnosis

A. Detection of antibody to HIV:
- ELISA (to detect antibody) is a sensitive test.
- Western Blot (to confirm HIV) is a confirmation test.

B. Virus isolation from cultured lymphocytes non-specific findings of HIV/AIDS:
- Anaemia
- Leucopenia (especially lymphocytopenia)
- Thrombocytopenia
- Polyclonal hypergammaglobulinemia

Most widely used marker is absolute CD4 lymphocyte count. As the count decreases, risk of opportunistic infection increases.

Control of AIDS: Prevention of blood borne HIV transmission: Advise people with high risk groups to avoid donating **blood, body organs, sperm or other tissues**.

All blood should be screened for HIV 1 and 2 before blood transfusion.

Transmission to hemophiliacs can be decreased by introducing heat treatment of factors VIII and IX.

Strict sterilization practices ensured in hospitals and clinics.

Pre-sterilized disposable syringes and needles should be used as much as possible. Avoid injections unless absolutely necessary.

Counselling of HIV positive patients

- Consult a clinician experienced in treating HIV/AIDS.
- Protect ex-partner(s) from HIV by following safe-sex guidelines.
- Inform sex partner(s) who may also be infected.

- Do not share needles.
- Get information and social and legal support from AIDS service organizations.
- Don't share HIV status with people who do not need to know. Only tell people you can count on for support. Think about whom do you want to share your HIV status with.
- Get psychological support from a counselor and/or join a support group for people with HIV.
- Maintain a strong immune system with a healthy lifestyle and regular medical examinations.
- Consider using anti-retroviral therapies that may slow the progress of the infection in consultation with a qualified physician.

HEPATITIS B AND HEPATITIS C VIRUS INFECTION

ELISA FOR HBsAg

- It is an in-*vitro* enzyme immunoassay.
- Specific monoclonal anti-HBs antibodies are used.
- It is **direct, non-competitive, solid phase enzyme immuno-assay** with horse radish peroxidase as the marker enzyme.
- HBsAg when present combines with mouse monoclonal anti-HBsAbs coated on the polystrene surface of the wells and simultaneously combines with horse radish peroxidase conjugated sheep poly and mouse monoclonal anti-HBs antibodies.
- After incubation washed colourless substrate and chromogen added.
- The enzyme action produces coloured end product.
- Reaction is terminated by stop solution (1.6N H_2SO_4).

Procedure ELISA for HBsAg Detection

Mix conjugate and conjugate diluent in the ratio of 1:26
- Sample 1 100 µl
- Sample 2 100 µl
- Sample 3 100 µl
  Run positive and negative controls.

25 µl conjugate to each well and mix, incubate for 60–90 min at 37°C. (According to Manual)

5–10 min before, mix substrate solution and substrate diluent 1:101. Wash the wells.

100 µl of substrate into all wells, incubate for 30 min at room temperature.

Add stop solution. Read the absorbance as per the instructions given by users manual. Positive or negative reading is given according to the cut-off value which is calculated as per the manufacture's manual.

NUCLEIC ACID TESTING (NAT)

- Nucleic acid testing (NAT) is used for the screening of human immunodeficiency virus, hepatitis B and hepatitis C virus in donated blood. This test is the first simultaneous, single tube NAT solution for HIV, HCV and HBV. It is a direct test where it actually detects the viral nucleic acid (RNA/DNA). Being a direct test it reduces the window period for detection for all these three viruses from the current available serological (ELISA) tests.[8]
- NAT combines the advantages of direct detection of the organism with sensitivity several orders of magnitude higher than that of traditional methods. The screening of blood for infectious markers (anti-HIV 1 and 2, anti-HCV and HBsAg) is done using government approved test kits (ELISA or rapid kits).
- Despite these efforts, residual risk of transfusion-transmitted infections remains because of donors in the pre-seroconversion (window period), viral variants, non-seroconverting (immunosilent) or delayed seroconverting carriers (atypical seroconversion).
- Nucleic acid testing (NAT) along with serological testing can reduce this residual risk to a great extent because it involves highly specific detection of an infectious agent (the virus itself) with much higher sensitivity.
- NAT is a recently developed technology that allows detection of very small amounts of genetic material (DNA or RNA) by a process of massive copying (amplification) of a gene fragment.

- Currently, donors of blood and plasma are tested for hepatitis B surface antigen, antibodies to HCV, antibodies to HIV and HIV antigens, which are the virus' own proteins.
- NAT has reduced the "window period" for detection of HBV to 10.34 days, HCV to 1.34 days and HIV to 2.93 days.[8]
- Given the high rate of sero-positivity of HIV, HCV and HBV in India and keeping in mind the high percentage of first time and replacement donors, it is likely that adding NAT to the current screening tests will have a very significant reduction in transfusion transmitted infections making transfusion of blood safer.

VDRL (SYPHILIS)

Blood is tested for syphilis by the following methods:
- Venereal diseases research laboratory (VDRL).
- *Treponema pallidum* haemagglutination assay (TPHA).
- Fluorescent treponemal antibody-absorbed test (FTA-abs).
- Enzyme immunoassay (EIA) tests.

Preservation of Blood, Principles and its Applications in Blood Banking

History

Before the era of preservative solutions, direct artery to vein blood transfusion was practiced.

In the year 1910, Fleig described the procedure of storage of red cells.

In 1914, Hustin transfused first citrated blood to humans and the safety of citrate was described.

In 1915, Weil found out a procedure and citrated blood was stored in a ice box.

In 1916, Rous and Turner used citrate sucrose solution, and later found that dextrose was better than sucrose. Rous and Turner's solution was used for storage of human blood during the First World War.

In 1937, the first modern blood bank was established in Cook County Hospital, Chicago by Benard Fantus as director and Oswald Robertson as an advisor.

In 1943, Loutit and Mollison introduced acidified citrate dextrose (ACD) solution. This solution was used during the Second World War for clinical use.

In 1957, Gibson *et al* developed citrate phosphate-dextrose (CPD) which is:

- Less acidic than ACD
- 2,3-diphosphoglycerate (2,3-DPG) levels are better in CPD than in ACD solution.
- CPD has eventually replaced ACD
- Shelf-life of blood stored in CPD at 2–4°C is 21 days.

In 1978, Nakao *et al* and Simon used citrate-phosphate-dextrose with adenine (CPDA-1). Addition of adenine improved the synthesis of adenosine triphosphate (ATP) in the stored blood, which prolonged the storage of blood/red cells at 2–4°C to 35 days.

PRESERVATIVES SOLUTIONS

Acid Citrate Dextrose (ACD)

Trisodium citrate	1.485 g
Citric acid	0.540 g
Dextrose	1.687 g

In a volume of 67.5 mL for 450 mL of blood.
pH after collection is 7.0, falls to 6.7 with storage. Shelf life is 21 days.

Citrate Phosphate Dextrose (CPD)

Trisodium citrate	1.66 g
Citric acid (monohydrate)	0.206 g
Sod. dihydrogen monophosphate	0.140 g
Dextrose	1.61 g

In a volume of 63 mL for 450 mL of blood.
Higher pH and phosphate enhances 2,3-DPG content.
pH 7.2 on day 0, falls to 6.8 during storage day 21. Shelf life is 21 days.

Citrate Phosphate Dextrose A-1 (CPDA-1)

Trisodium citrate	1.66 g
Citric acid (monohydrate)	0.206 g
Sod. dihydrogen monophosphate	0.140 g
Dextrose	2.01 g
Adenine (0.25 mM)	0 .017 g

In a volume of 63 mL for 450 mL of blood, shelf life is 35 days.

Action of Ingredients of Anticoagulant Solutions

Dextrose: Supports ATP generation by glycolytic pathways and prevents lysis of cells.

Adenine: Synthesizes ATP, extends shelf life of red cells to 35 days.

Citrate: Prevents coagulation by chelating calcium.

Sodium diphosphate: Prevents fall in pH.

Changes occurring with stored blood are the following:
- **Loss of red cell viability is due to:**
  – Decrease in pH
  – Built up of lactic acid
  – Decrease in glucose
  – Decrease in ATP level
  – Low 2,3 DPG levels
- **Red cell preservation:** The goal of blood preservation is to provide viable and functional blood components for patients requiring blood transfusion.

  More than 70% of red cells should remain viable in circulation 24 hours after transfusion of stored blood in CPDA-1 for 35 days.

  The blood is stored at 2–6°C to maintain the optimal viability.
- **pH changes:** When blood is stored at 2–6°C, glycolysis is reduced but does not stop.

  Glycolysis results in the production of lactate with subsequent decrease in pH.

  Whole blood collected in CPD has a pH of 7.2 on day 0 and 6.84 on day 21.

  Preservative solutions provide buffering capability to minimize pH changes and optimize the storage period.
- **Adenosine triphosphate (ATP):** ATP is associated with the red cells viability.

  Loss of ATP causes increase in cellular rigidity and decrease in red cell membrane integrity and deformability.

  Decrease in ATP allows the leak of Na^+ and K^+ through the red cell membrane at levels exceeding those normally seen *in vivo*. The ATP level in CPDA-1 red cells at day 35 is 45% ($\pm$12) of the initial level.
- **2,3-diphosphoglycerate (2,3-DPG):** With fall in pH, red cell 2,3-DPG level decreases which increases haemoglobin-oxygen affinity.

DPG-depleted red cells have impaired capacity to deliver oxygen to the tissues.

The degree of reduction of 2,3-DPG levels depends upon the preservative solution used.

ACD solution has lower pH than that of CPD solution.

Thus 2,3-DPG falls within the first few days in ACD, whereas blood stored in CPD/CPDA-1 maintains adequate levels of 2,3-DPG for 10–14 days.

- **After transfusion, the red cells continue to synthesize ATP.** 2,3-DPG levels return to expected normal values within 24 hours.

  2,3-DPG levels in transfused blood are important in certain clinical conditions.

  The pathological effects of low 2,3-DPG levels with increased affinity with oxygen increases cardiac output.

  Myocardial function improves with transfusion of blood high in 2,3-DPG levels during cardiovascular surgery.

  In patients with shock, the transfusion of 2,3-DPG-depleted red cells makes a significant difference in recovery.

- **Adenine:** CPD solution supplemented with 17 mg (0.25 mm) adenine per 63 mL of anticoagulant and 25% more dextrose, the survival of red cells 24 hours after transfusion of blood stored for 35 days may be around 80%.

  Adenine synthesizes ATP and its level is 56.4 ± 15.9% of the initial level in the stored blood for five weeks.

  Adenine causes nephrotoxicity due to its unmetabolized product, 2,8-dioxyadenine, however, toxicity is negligible with 15 mg/kg body weight.

- **Changes in Na$^+$ and K$^+$ levels:** During storage, Na$^+$ and K$^+$ leak through the red cell membrane rapidly. The cells loose K$^+$ and gain Na$^+$, however, the K$^+$ loss is greater than the Na$^+$ gain during storage.

- **Temperature:** The lower temperature keeps the rate of glycolysis at lower limit and minimizes the proliferation of bacteria that might have entered the blood unit during venipuncture or from atmosphere. The rate of diffusion of electrolytes (Na$^+$ and K$^+$) across the cell membrane is also less at a lower temperature.

- **Heparin:** Heparin prevents coagulation by inactivating the prophylactic activity of thrombin after complexing with antithrombin III.

  Dose of heparin for anticoagulation is 0.5–2.0 IU/mL of blood, e.g. approximately 500 IU of heparin for 500 mL of blood. Heparinized blood should be used within 24 hours.

Additive Solutions

Additive solutions were discovered in 1983. This system has a primary bag containing CPD and a satellite bag containing 100 ml of additive solution. The additive solution is added to only red cells, as only they are benefited with this procedure. Plasma and platelets are separated first. The additive solution is added to the remaining red cells within 72 hours of phlebotomy. With this procedure:

- Shelf life of RBCs is extended to 42 days
- ATP levels are maintained

Following are the additive solutions which are in use:

- SAG, SAGM/SAGMAN (saline, adenine, glucose, mannitol)
- Adsol (AS-1)
- Nutricel (AS-3)
- Optisol (AS-5).

  Composition of some of the additive solutions is given below.

Additive solution AS-1

Dextrose	2.20 g
Adenine (0.25 mM)	27 mg
Mannitol	750 mg
Sodium chloride	900 mg
In a volume of 100 mL	

Additive solution AS-3

Trisodium citrate	588 mg
Sod. dihydrogen monophosphate	276 mg
Citric acid (monohydrate)	42 mg
Dextrose	1.10 g
Adenine (0.25 mM)	30 mg
Mannitol	—
Sodium chloride	410 mg
In a volume of 100 mL	

Additive solution AS-5

Trisodium citrate	—
Sod. dihydrogen monophosphate	—
Citric acid (monohydrate)	—
Dextrose	900 mg
Adenine (0.25 mM)	30 mg
Mannitol	525 mg
Sod. chloride	877 mg
In a volume of 100 mL	

SAGM is the currently used additive solution in Europe. AS-1, AS-5 and AS-3 are now licensed in USA.[9]

Rejuvenate Solutions

To increase the levels of 2,3-DPG and ATP in stored blood, rejuvenation solution can be added. These solutions:
- Have phosphate, inosine, glucose, pyruvate and adenine.
- Increase the levels of 2,3-DPG and ATP.
- Solution added at any time after 3 days collection up to 3 days after expiration of shelf life.
- Rejuvenation solution is added to red blood cells, incubated for 1 hr and washed.
- 50 mL sterile solution (rejuvenol, cytosol laboratories, braintree, MA) is commercially available.
- The rejuvenation process is expensive and time consuming and is rarely used.
  Note: For composition of rejuvenol, refer to topic on blood and blood components.

Plastic Bags

- Many other factors may limit the viability of transfused red cells. One of the factors is also the plastic material used for the bags.
- The plastic material should be sufficiently permeable to CO_2 in order to maintain higher pH during storage. If not removed at a controlled rate, the pH value of the blood is reduced which shortens the life of blood components.
- Blood is stored in plastic bags made of polyvinyl chloride (PVC) with plasticizer, di-(2-ethylhexyl) phthalate (DEHP).

- New plastic bags made of polyolefin with new plasticizer (Baxter's PL 732) and thin walled PVC with tri-(2-ethylhexyl) trimellate plasticizer (TOTM) [Baxter's PL 1240 and Cutter CLX] are available with higher permeability of gases (O_2 and CO_2) and platelets can be stored for 5 days.

Red Cell Freezing

Freezing damages red cells due to the intracellular ice formation and to some extent due to hypertonicity.

Red cells mixed with glycerol could be frozen without damage.

If glycerol (cryoprotective agent) is added to the cells, they can be frozen and thawed without damage.

The effect of the glycerol is probably due to the fact that it limits ice formation and provides liquid phase in which salts are distributed. As cooling proceeds, excessive hypertonicity is also avoided.

The cells are rapidly frozen and stored in a freezer. The freezing and storage temperature depends on the concentration of glycerol.

Frozen red cells are used in autologous transfusion and the storage of blood with rare blood groups.

Two concentrations are used to freeze red cells, a high concentration glycerol 40% weight in volume (w/v) and a low concentration glycerol 20% weight in volume (w/v).

Most blood banks use the high glycerol technique.

Platelet Preservation

The preservation of viable and functional platelets depends on the following factors:

- **Temperature:** Platelets should be stored at 22–24°C (controlled temperature) with continuous gentle agitation in platelet incubator and agitator.
- **pH:** pH should be above 6.0.
- **Plastic bag:** Maintenance of pH and function of platelets depend on the permeability of the storage bag to oxygen and carbon dioxide.
- Platelets stored in bags made of polyvinyl chloride (PVC) with plasticizer di-(2-ethylhexyl) phthalate (DEHP) have shelf life of 3 days.

- New plastic bags maintain pH and function up to about 7 days. However, it is recommended to store platelets for 5 days only from the date of collection.

Granulocyte Preservation

- The shelf life of granulocytes is 24 hours at 22–24°C. They do not need agitation.
- Post-transfusion recovery of granulocytes in circulation and migration into inflammatory site is better if transfused within 8 hours of storage than that of granulocytes stored for 24 hours.

Fresh Frozen Plasma (FFP)

Shelf life of FFP is 12 months at –18°C or lower. After thawing, FFP can be stored at 2–6°C for 6 hours before transfusion. FFP contains plasma proteins and all coagulation factors including factor VIII.

Recovered Plasma

Recovered plasma is plasma that can be separated from donors red cells at any time up to 5 days after the expiration of blood. This contains all stable coagulation factors including fibrinogen and factor IX. For details refer to topic on "Blood and Blood Components".

Cryoprecipitate

Cryoprecipitate can be stored for 12 months at –18°C or lower. Thawed cryoprecipitate can be stored for 6 hours at 2–6°C and pooled cryoprecipitate kept at 2–6°C should be used within 6 hours. For details refer to topic on "Blood and Blood Components".

Transporting Blood and Blood Components within the Hospital

- The blood and red cells should be transported within the hospital in insulated carrier or in cold insulated boxes if the ambient temperature is more than 25°C.
- Instructions should be given to keep the blood bag in the blood bank refrigerator if there is possibility that blood/red cells will not be transfused immediately.

Transporting platelets: Transporting of stored platelets to the transfusion facility should use a well-insulated container, with no ice, to maintain the temperature between 20° and 24°C.

Transporting of frozen components

- Fresh frozen plasma and cryoprecipitate must be transported at –18°C or below.
- Dry ice is used to maintain the frozen state. Dry ice should be kept at the bottom and at the top of the well-insulated container.
- Check breakage during transportation.

Storage of Blood

- Temperature range: 2°–6°C except for platelets with a temperature range of 22°–24°C.
- Refrigerator for storing blood should have a fan for circulating air to ensure uniform temperature.
- System should be there to monitor and record the temperature continuously.
- Temperature recording charts should be changed regularly.
- There should be alarms.
- In case where blood has to be transported (camps), blood should be packed in cold boxes surrounded by ice packs.

Advantages of lower temperature

- Keeps the rate of glycolysis at a lower limit.
- Minimizes the proliferation of bacteria.
- Reduces the rate of diffusion of electrolytes (Na and K) across the cell membrane.
- Blood should be administered within half an hour of receiving from the blood bank.

General Requirements for Storage of Blood and Blood Products

- The anticoagulant/preservative solutions with proper temperature are essential for maintaining the viability and stability of the blood and its products.
- Separate areas should be reserved for storing untested and tested products.
- No food should be stored in the refrigerators and freezers.

Blood and Blood Components

GOALS OF BLOOD TRANSFUSION

The goal of transfusion medicine is to provide the safest and the most appropriate blood product for the patient to meet the desired outcome.

The transfusion should:

i. Aid the patient to improve his/her condition.

ii. The transfusion should have more benefits than the potential risks.

The major indications for the transfusion of blood or blood products are to restore or maintain the following:

1. Blood volume
2. Oxygen carrying capacity of blood
3. Hemostasis and
4. Leucocytic function

A patient's clinical condition is the most important factor to consider when determining the transfusion needs of the patient. Once it has been determined that transfusion is necessary, then it becomes crucial to ascertain which blood product or products will best serve the needs of the patient.

A variety of components are available. With component therapy many patients can benefit from the blood drawn from one donor.

The reasons for separation of blood components are as follows:

• From whole blood various components can be prepared. Whole blood storage conditions are not optimal for all functional components of blood. For example, after 24 hours of storage at 1° to 6°C whole blood has a few viable platelets and granulocytes. Stable coagulation factors are well maintained during storage, but heat labile factors like factor V and VIII decrease with time and may not be adequate to correct specific deficiencies in patients. The separation of various components allows storage of each component at the temperature and storage conditions required for *in vitro* survival.

- Component preparation allows transfusion of specific portion of blood product that the patient requires.
- Transfusion of required components avoids use of unnecessary whole blood transfusion which could be contra-indicated in some conditions. For example, risk of hyper-volemia in an elderly anaemic patient with congestive cardiac failure may not tolerate the transfusion of two units of whole blood.
- Also whole blood exposes to unnecessary antibodies. It also has white blood cells and platelets which can carry HLA antigens and can stimulate the patient's immune system.

PRINCIPLES OF COMPONENT PREPARATION

Component preparation programs must incorporate the principles of aseptic techniques using sterile, pyrogen-free equipment and solutions. Blood bags used for phlebotomy have integral, sterile extra bags known as **satellite bags** attached to the main collection bag. Approximately 450 mL of blood with 63 mL of anticoagulant is collected. Selected components can be transferred into the satellite bags through a closed system of tubing. The original phlebotomy bag may have one, two or three satellite bags attached. In the preparation of all compo-nents, sterility has to be assured. A break in the seal of a product at 20° to 24°C requires to be used within 4 hours.

Component preparation and separation is based on the principle that **different components** of whole blood have **different specific gravities**. For example, **red cells** represent the heaviest portion of whole blood with a **specific gravity of 1.08 to 1.09,** whereas **platelets** range between **1.03 and 1.04**. Using differential centrifugation with light spin of donated blood, the components separate into layers in the blood bag. The heaviest component settles to the bottom. In a unit of whole blood, the centrifuged products settle out in the following layers, starting from the bottom of the layer: Red blood cells, white blood cells and platelet-rich plasma (PRP). After separating the red cells from PRP, the plasma is centrifuged again for a longer time and at a harder (heavy) spin. This time the platelets settle at the bottom of the bag. The plasma is drawn off into the sterile connected bag with the platelets remaining in the first bag.

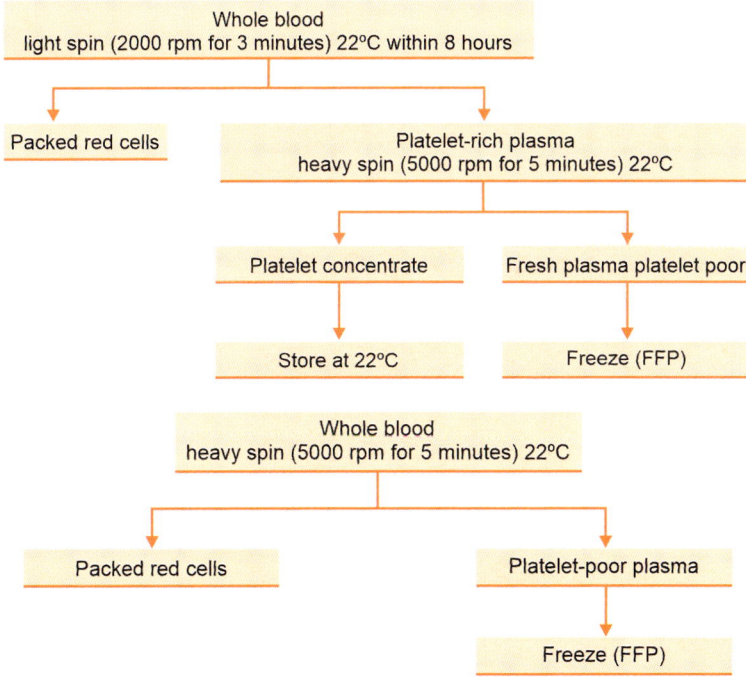

It is possible to make components with closed system or open system. Components prepared open system carry an increased risk of bacterial contamination.

Components containing red cells are the following:
- Unmodified stored whole blood
- Fresh blood

- Packed red blood cells (concentrated red cell suspension/PRBC)
- Optimal additive red cell suspensions
- Leucocyte poor/depleted red cells
- Deglycerolized red blood cells
- Rejuvenated red cells

Unmodified Stored Whole Blood

The approximate volume of each pack is 400–500 mL (450 with 63 mL of anticoagulant or 300 with 49 mL anticoagulant). Stored whole blood provides both plasma proteins and red cells. With storage there is decline in oxygen carrying capacity, but this reaches normal levels within 24–48 hours following transfusion. **Labile factors, principally factor V and factor VIII, will also be reduced. Functional platelets and granulocytes are absent but their antigenic residues are present.**

Stored whole blood was often used in earlier days. With increased demand for blood components have now reduced its use.

Indications whole blood

- Massive blood transfusion
- Exchange transfusion

Fresh Blood

Fresh blood that is collected within the preceding 24 hours provides volume, red blood cells with normal oxygen affinity, coagulation factors and platelets. Potassium levels are in normal levels, whereas they are elevated in stored blood. In conditions where platelets are of paramount importance, blood has to be transfused soon after collection and certainly prior to refrigeration.

Special requests for fresh blood may be received on occasion for selected patients such as neonatal patient. Newborns are sometimes candidates for fresh blood because newborn has a high percentage of fetal haemoglobin which does not release oxygen to the tissues.

The levels of 2,3-diphosphoglycerate may be decreased in certain conditions such as respiratory distress syndrome. Using the same rationale, an **exchange transfusion** is another procedure in which it is appropriate to use blood of less than seven days old.

Red Cells Suspensions (Packed Red Blood Cells)

Packed red cells are prepared by removing most of the plasma from a unit of whole blood. Since red cells have a higher specific gravity than plasma, they move to lower portion of the collection bag by either gravitational settling or centrifugation. Then this plasma portion is removed from top of the bag into a satellite bag. This plasma portion may be used for further component preparation.

These red cells packs are named with anticoagulant or preservative used in the primary bags. For example, if anti-coagulant CPDA-1 is used, the red blood cell product is labeled as CPDA-1 red blood cells. All anticoagulants and preservatives solution used for whole blood are approved for red cells except heparin. Heparin is used for whole blood only. Red blood cells have an approximate volume of 300 mL. The final haematocrit of packed cells should not exceed 80% (range 0.65–0.75) and should be stored at temperature of 1° to 6°C.

Red cells packs are used for:

- Patients with symptomatic anaemia because they provide needed oxygen carrying capacity without unnecessary volume.
- Red cells may also be used for newborn exchange trans-fusion. In these patients the unit should be less than 7 days old to avoid problem associated with increased potassium levels in the neonate and to ensure maximum 2, 3-DPG levels.
- Red cells packs can be used in surgeries.

Optimal Additive Red Cells Suspensions

These are red cells packs to which around 100 mL of a nutrient preservative solution have been added. They are used under the same circumstances as red cells. The lower haematocrit permits faster infusion flow rate. For details refer to topic on "preservation of blood, principles and its applications in blood banking".

Leucocyte-depleted (Reduced) Red Cells

Leucocytes in blood products can induce adverse reaction in sensitized patient. These side effects include **non-haemolytic febrile transfusion reaction (NHFTR) which is caused by allo-immunisation of the patient to foreign human leucocyte antigens (HLA).**

Leucocyte deduction can effectively reduce the incidence of these adverse reactions and can also reduce the risk of transmission of certain viral infection that are primarily found in leucocytes, e.g. CMV, EBV and HTLV-1.

Leucocyte reduced red cells can be used:
- Prophylactically to reduce the risk of allo-immunisation to HLA antigens in transplant patients.
- In patients with long-term multi-transfusion therapy to avoid non-haemolytic febrile reactions.

Methods of preparation of leucocyte reduced red cell products include the following:
- Centrifugation
- Saline washing
- Spin-cool-filtration
- Freezing and deglycerolization
- Bedside filtration
- Pre-storage filtration

In the **centrifugation method of leucocyte reduction**, the buffy coat layer between the red cells and plasma is drawn off into a satellite bag, along with some of the red cells. The same procedure can be followed in inverted position. The red cells are drained into satellite bag, leaving the leucocyte and plasma in the primary bag. Although this is a simple and cost effective technique, when compared with other techniques the leucocyte reduction is only 70–80% of the original number. Up to 20% of the red cells are lost by this procedure.

Washing of red cells removes leucocytes and plasma. This removes 70–95% of leucocytes and 14–15% of red cells. The washed cells have an expiration time of 24 hours. This method of leucocyte reduction is comparatively expensive owing to the washing equipment and special bags required.

The **spin-cool-filter method** removes approximately 90% leucocytes. Less than 10% of red cells are removed. The red cells are centrifuged at 1° to 6°C in an inverted position, placed in 4°C storage for 3 hours and then filtered using a standard micro-aggregate filter prior to infusion at the bedside. The centrifugation brings the white cells together in the buffy coat layer, the cooling further aggregates the white cells and the micro-aggregate filter removes the leucocyte aggregates. Although this procedure is labour intensive, it is cost effective and simple.

Red cells can be **frozen in glycerolized** state and later thawed and deglycerolized. The deglycerolized red cells have leucocyte reduction in the range of 95–99% but have a red cell loss of 20%. To get deglycerolized red cells for leucocyte reduction is an expensive procedure. Once the product is thawed, the shelf life is only for 24 hours.

Leucocyte reduction can be achieved with use of **leucocyte depletion filters** at the **patient's bedside**. Leucocyte reduction filters are used during infusion in place of standard blood filter. Leucocyte reduction filters reduce leucocytes in the product by 99% and allow greater than 90% of the red blood cells to be transfused.

Pre-storage filtration for leucocyte reduction: Leucocytes begin to disintegrate quickly when stored at 1° to 6°C. These white cell fragments may be capable of initiating an immune response to HLA antigens and also can release cytokines and chemical mediators like histamine and causes FNHTR. In order to prevent the fragmentation of leucocytes, it may be desirable to remove white cells before storage using a sterile connection device or in-line filter. The donor's red cells are filtered within 8 hours of phlebotomy.

Deglycerolized/Frozen Red Blood Cells

Red cells are frozen in glycerolized state and thawed and deglycerolized. Frozen red cells are prepared for various reasons which may include: (1) Storage of blood from a rare donor and (2) Autologous units for future scheduled surgery.

The red cells from a whole blood are separated and **frozen within 6 days of donation**. Freezing allows extended storage up to 10 years from the date of original phlebotomy.

Freezing of red cells requires the addition of cryoprotective agent prior to freezing to prevent cellular damage or haemolysis. To provide maximum protection, an optimal balance between cellular dehydration and intracellular ice crystal formation must be achieved. The basic methods for cryoprecipitate are: (1) High glycerol, (2) low glycerol and (3) agglomeration. High glycerol is used by most of the organizations. In this method, the red cells are prepared for cryopreservation by the addition of 6.2 M glycerol to the red cells. The final concentration of glycerol is 40% weight of solute per volume solution (w/v), with approximately 400 mL of 6.2 M glycerol added to the red cells. The process is done in two steps allowing gradual equilibration of the glycerol in the red cells. For best results red cells and glycerol are mixed at room temperature to allow diffusion of glycerol into the cells. Then the red cells are frozen at –80°C and stored at –65°C. For deglycerolization, the cryoprotective glycerol must be slowly removed and replaced with isotonic solution before transfusion to the patient. Frozen red cells, once deglycerolized are stored at 1° to 6°C. Once the product is thawed, the shelf life is only 24 hours from the time the red cell bag was entered for deglycerolization.

Rejuvenated Red Cells

Red cells stored at 1° to 6°C, continuously loose both 2,3-DPG and adenosine triphosphate (ATP). The level of 2,3-DPG correlates with the ability of the red cells to deliver oxygen to the tissues. The viability of the red cells correlates with ATP levels. After transfusion, the levels of both 2, 3-DPG and ATP return to normal in the patient within 24 hours of transfusion. It is possible to restore the levels *in vitro* prior to transfusion by the use of rejuvenation solution, e.g. REJUVENOL. Ingredients of REJUVENOL in 50 mL of sterile pyrogen-free water with pH 6.7 to 7.4 is given below:

Sodium pyruvate	550 mg
Inosine	34 mg
Dibasic sodium phosphate	500 mg
Monobasic sodium phosphate	200 mg

The red cells are to be incubated with the rejuvenating solution at 37°C for 1 hour. Only red cells can be rejuvenated. Once the red cells are rejuvenated, they must be washed before transfusion and used within 24 hours. Rejuvenation is an expensive process. However, it is an excellent tool for preserving rare units of blood.

Platelet Preparations

Platelets are required for treatment of thrombocytopenic patients, who are judged to be at risk of haemorrhagic symptoms.

Platelets are required in haematological malignancies, particularly in acute myeloid leukemia. Platelets are valuable in the treatment of acute self-limiting conditions or for isolated bleeding episodes. In chronic states long-term blood transfusion or platelet therapy is inevitable as it leads to allo-immunisation against broad range of HLA or platelet-specific antigens. This complication seriously diminishes the chances of providing serologically compatible and clinically effective therapy.

The risk of bleeding is greater with falling counts than with rising counts. Platelet counts below $10 \times 10^9/L$ are at high risk and patients who are not showing thrombocytopenic symptoms may need prophylactic therapy. **Patients with symptoms and those requiring surgery with platelet counts ranging between $20–50 \times 10^9/L$ platelets should be transfused**.

Volume: 150–300 mL.

Unit of issue: SDP (1 therapeutic dose), has approximately **$3.5–4 \times 10^{11}$** platelets RDP (4–6 units—1 therapeutic dose), one unit of RDP has average $5.5–7.5 \times 10^{10}$ of platelets.

Infection risk: Same as whole blood.

RDP exposes to 4–6 donors and has chances of bacterial infection.

Dosage: 1 unit of RDP/10 kg body wt. or 1 SDP.

Storage: 5 days at 22–24°C with agitation.

Not to be refrigerated.

Administration: Compatible donor required.

Precautions: Febrile transfusion reaction, allergic reactions.

Acute transfusion reactions because of bacterial contamination.

Fresh Frozen Plasma and Related Products

One unit of plasma is obtained from centrifugation of one unit of whole blood and usually contains 180–300 mL. When obtained from single donor from plasmapheresis the amount of plasma obtained is two to three times more than that obtained from whole blood, i.e. **500 to 800 mL.** When plasma is stored at –20°C within 6 hours of collection is called fresh frozen plasma (FFP). Cryo-poor or cryo-supernatant plasma is the plasma product which remains after obtaining cryoprecipitate fraction from FFP through cold precipitation.

Single donor plasma (source plasma) is stored at –20°C within 6 hours of collection.

Plasma from whole blood obtained within 5 days of expiration date of whole of blood is called recovered plasma.

Unit of issue: Usual pack of 200–300 mL.

Smaller volume packs for children.

Infection risk: Same as whole blood.

Storage: One year at –20°C.

Before use, thawed at 30–37°C, higher temperature will destroy clotting factors and plasma proteins.

Precautions: Acute allergic reactions, especially with rapid infusions anaphylactic reactions occasionally occur hypovolaemia alone is not an indication of use.

Dosage: Initial dose of 15 mL/kg.

FFP once collected from the blood bank can be preserved at 1–6°C and has to be used within 6 hours.

Cryoprecipitate

One unit of cryoprecipitate is defined as that obtained from a single FFP bag.

Procedure for preparation of cryoprecipitate: Thaw FFP at 1 to 6°C. Precipitate will be formed at the bottom of the sterile bag. This precipitate portion is re-suspended in 5–10 mL of plasma and re-frozen within 1 hour and stored at –18°C. This can be stored for 1 year.

Cryoprecipitate has:
- Factor VIII (80–100 U)
- von Willebrand's factor (80 U of the original plasma concentration)
- Fibrinogen (100–250 mg)
- Fibronectin (50–60 mg)
- Factor XIII (40–60 U of the original plasma concentration)

The half life of factor VIII is 8–12 hours, so transfusion of factor VIII is repeated every 8–12 hours. Cryoprecipitate is thawed to 37°C before transfusion and administered through standard blood filter. No compatibility testing is needed. It has to be used within 6 hours of thawing.

Unit of issue: Single donor pack/6 or more packs of single donor units pooled.

Infection risk: Same as plasma.

Administration: If possible ABO compatible.

No compatibility testing required.

Blood Transfusion in Clinical Practice

Indications for Red Cell Transfusion

- While defining indications for red cell transfusion, one cannot base it only on the values of haemoglobin (Hb) and haematocrit (Ht). Firstly, one has to evaluate patient's age, nature of disease and co-morbidities, expected surgical procedures, coagulation abnormalities, the amount of blood expected to be lost because of bleeding, clinical and physiological parameters, showing an overall condition of a patient and tolerance to an expected tissue hypoxemia due to anaemia.
- What is more, one must take into consideration is body temperature, heart function, heart rate, arterial blood pressure, renal function, venous blood oxygen saturation, and blood oxygen partial pressure.
- The main indication for **red cell transfusion is to keep adequate oxygen-carrying capacity of blood and to avoid or reduce tissue hypoxia. The red cell transfusion should not be done only to increase the Hb level** (except the cases of severe symptoms of anaemia and the need to ameliorate the oxygen-carrying capacity).
- In case of anaemia, the delivery of oxygen is ameliorated by physiological adaptability mechanisms: The haemoglobin affinity for oxygen decreases, oxygen-haemoglobin dissociation curve shifts to right, oxygen release from red cells increases, peripheral vascular resistance and blood viscosity decrease; furthermore, the cardiac output increases due to increased heart rate, stroke volume and contractility.

- The consumption of oxygen depends on these factors like physical activity, body temperature, sympathetic and metabolic activity, heart rate, and the effect of certain drugs (e.g. anaesthetics).
- Young and healthy women without hypovolemia can tolerate acute anaemia quite well. The delivery of oxygen remains adequate, and there may not be severe symptoms of anaemia even though Hb concentration decreases to 6 g/dL.
- When treating major haemorrhage, firstly, the volume of lost blood should be estimated. **The goal of maintaining adequate tissue perfusion is normovolemia; therefore, one of the main principles in treating acute bleeding is to restore circulating blood volume by fluids, but not by red cell transfusion.** PCV/Hb **should not** be considered as the only laboratory markers when estimating bleeding level, because these markers can be influenced by the initial infusion therapy.[10]
- The average adult blood volume represents 7% of body weight (or 70 mL/kg of body weight). Estimated blood volume (EBV) for a 70 kg person is approximately 5 litres. Blood volume varies with age and physiologic state. Older individuals have a smaller blood volume. Children have EBVs of 8–9% of body weight, with infants having an EBV as high as 9–10% of their total body weight.[11]

Blood Transfusion in Anaemia

In chronic anaemias, red cell transfusion is given according to the Hb level which is given below:

- **Hb >10 g/dL**, if patient's condition is stable—no indication for red cell transfusion.
- **Hb <6 g/dL**, transfusion almost always indicated.
- **Hb 6–10 g/dL**, indication for transfusion is based on any ongoing indication of organ ischemia, the rate and magnitude of any potential or actual bleeding, the patient's intravascular volume status and risk of complications due to inadequate oxygenation.
- **When Hb level is less than 7 g/dL and anaemia is asymptomatic**, transfusion is needed **if massive bleeding is expected during surgery** or the patient belongs to a high anaesthetic risk group.

The AABB guidelines include the following recommendations.[12]

- Hb <6 g/dL: Transfusion recommended except in exceptional cases.
- Hb 6 to 7 g/dL: Transfusion generally likely to be indicated.
- Hb 7 to 8 g/dL: Transfusion in postoperative cases.
- Hb 8 to 10 g/dL: Transfusion generally not indicated except in exceptional cases (e.g. ongoing bleeding, acute coronary syndrome with ischemia, etc.).
- Hb >10 g/dL: Transfusion generally not indicated except in exceptional cases.

According to Kenyan Government, 2004 Guidelines for the Appropriate Use of Blood and Blood Products[13] is given below.

- Red cell transfusion is rarely indicated when haemoglobin levels are greater than 10 gm/dL, and is usually indicated when haemoglobin concentrations are less than 5 gm/dL. However, even severely anaemic patients (less than 5 gm/dL Hb) who are clinically stable may not require transfusion.
- Transfuse only to decrease symptoms and to minimize risk (generally at Hb of less than 5 gm/dL). Do not transfuse above 5 gm/dL Hb unless patient is symptomatic.
- Treat nutritional and mild blood loss anaemia with specific therapeutic agents as indicated (iron, folic acid, B12).

  Use specific strategies for sickle cell disease and thalassemia.

One unit of donor erythrocytes (around 250 mL), the usage of blood components in a 70 kg patient increases Hb by about 1 g/dL and PCV by 3%.

A unit of whole blood has a volume of approximately **400 to 500 mL**, with a haematocrit **of 45 to 55%**. A unit of PRBCs consists of the red blood cells concentrated from a unit of whole blood. Each unit of PRBCs contains approximately **180 to 200 mL of RBCs and 50 to 70 mL of plasma**. The **haematocrit of PRBCs is 65 to 75%**.

Red cell transfusion in blood loss

- **Loss of <15%** of **circulating blood volume** (CBV) (up to **750 mL): No need to transfuse red cells,** unless anaemia or severe heart or pulmonary diseases were diagnosed before haemorrhage.

- **Loss of 15–30%** of CBV (around 750–1500 mL): **Crystalloids and synthetic colloids** should be given; usually there is no need for red cell transfusion, unless anaemia or severe heart or pulmonary disease is diagnosed and the bleeding continues.
- **Loss of 30–40%** of CBV (around **1500–2000** mL): Hypovolemia is corrected by crystalloids and synthetic colloids and red cell transfusion is usually indicated.
- **Loss of >40%** of CBV (**>2000 mL**): Urgent correction of hypovolemia, including red cell transfusion, must be performed.

Haemorrhage is broken down into four classes by the American College of Surgeons.[14]

- **Class I Haemorrhage** involves up to 15% of blood volume. There is typically no change in vital signs and fluid resuscitation is not usually necessary.
- **Class II Haemorrhage** involves 15–30% of total blood volume. A patient is often tachycardic (rapid heart beat) with a narrowing of the difference between the systolic and diastolic blood pressures. The body attempts to compensate with peripheral vasoconstriction. Skin may look pale and be cool to the touch. The patient may exhibit slight changes in behavior. Volume resuscitation with crystalloids (saline or Ringer's lactate) is all that is required. Blood transfusion is not typically required.
- **Class III Haemorrhage** involves loss of 30–40% of circulating blood volume. The patient's blood pressure drops, the heart rate increases, peripheral hypoperfusion (shock) and the mental status worsen. **Volume correction with crystalloid and blood transfusion** are usually necessary.
- **Class IV Haemorrhage** involves loss of >40% of circulating blood volume. The limit of the body's compensation is reached and **aggressive volume correction** is required to prevent death.
- As a general rule, less than 15% loss of blood volume results in minimal symptoms; 15 to 30% results in tachycardia; 30 to 40% in signs of shock; and greater than 40% in signs of severe shock. Some patients with underlying diseases may

require transfusion at 30 to 40% blood loss. Almost all patients require transfusion with losses greater than this.

Massive Haemorrhage

Blood loss is considered massive if:
- All blood volume is lost within a 24-hour period. (Normal blood volume in the adult is approximately 7% of ideal body weight); or
- 50% blood volume loss within 3 hours; or
- A rate of loss of 150 mL/minute.

Management of massive blood loss
- Aggressive **volume correction with colloids/crystalloids** (normal saline, Ringer's lactate, dextrose).
- A combination of packed red cells, FFP and platelets are indicated in 1:1:1 proportion. One proportion of platelets is one therapeutic dose (4–6 units of RDPs) or one pack of SDP.
- FFP and cryoprecipitate ideally be of the same blood group as that of the recipient.

Ways to minimize blood loss in massive haemorrhage
- Use of antifibrinolytic drugs
  - Tranexamic acid (orthopedic and cardiac surgeries)
  - Alprotinin
- Thrombo-elastography: Assesses dynamics of clot function, clot aggregation, clot strength and stability of clot.
- Protamine in place of low molecular weight heparin.
- Recombinant VIIa can be given.
- Desmopressin can be used to release factor VIII and vWF.

Other Guidelines for Red Cell Transfusion

Transfusion guidelines from College of American Pathologists (CAP)[15]

Target population: General.

RBC transfusion with following:
1. Hb <6 g/dL: Usually indicated.
2. Hb >10 g/dL: Rarely indicated.

3. Hb 6–10 g/dL: Decision depends upon extent of blood loss.
4. Previously healthy patients do not usually need transfusion even with losing 30–40% of their total blood volume and volume loss should be replaced by crystalloids and colloids RBC transfusion.
5. Transfusion decision should be made on peripheral tissue oxygenation, clinical signs and symptoms, Hb and extent and rate of bleeding.

Transfusion guidelines from American Society of Anaesthesiologists (ASA)[16]

In perioperative setting RBC transfusion is usually indicated as shown below.

1. In otherwise healthy individuals if Hb <6 g/dL.
2. Rarely indicated with Hb >10 g/dL.
3. In patients with Hb 6–10 g/dL with evidence of organ ischemia, rate and amount of bleeding, intravascular volume status and risk factors for inadequate oxygenation (e.g. low cardiopulmonary reserve) should be considered.

Transfusion guidelines from Society of Thoracic Surgeons and Society of Cardiovascular Anaesthesiologists (STS/SCA)[17]

In general cardiology surgery patients, RBC transfusions are considered:

1. To be reasonable if Hb <6 g/dL.
2. To be reasonable in most postoperative patients if Hb <7 g/dL.
3. May not be unreasonable in certain patients with Hb <10 g/dL in the presence of critical ischemia in other organs (e.g. central nervous system).
4. Rarely indicated if Hb >10 g/dL.

In patients undergoing cardiopulmonary bypass:

1. RBC transfusion is considered reasonable if Hb <6 g/dL.
2. May not be unreasonable to maintain Hb >7 g/dL in patients with risk of critical end organ ischemia.
3. Patient related factors like age, severity of illness, cardiac function, end organ ischemia, extent of blood loss, oxygen saturation, evidence of myocardial ischemia and other relevant parameters should be considered while decision making on RBC transfusion.

Transfusion guidelines from Society of Critical Care Medicine[18]

1. These guidelines are specifically for critically ill patients. RBC transfusions usually indicated with Hb <7 g/dL for patients requiring ventilation, critically ill trauma patients and patients with stable cardiac disease.
2. With Hb <8 g/dL in acute coronary syndrome, RBC transfusion may be beneficial.
3. Rarely indicated if Hb >10 g/dL.
4. Volume status, evidence of shock, duration/extent of anaemia cardiopulmonary parameters are considered while decision making on RBC transfusion.

Transfusion guidelines from the American Association of Blood Banks[19]

These guidelines are for hospitalized haemodynamically stable adult and children.

1. RBCs transfusions usually considered if Hb <7 g/dL for critically ill patients and Hb of 8 g/dL or <8 g/dL for patients undergoing surgery.
2. Hb levels and presence of symptoms are considered for decision making on RBC transfusion.

Transfusion of Platelets

Indications of platelet transfusion are given below:

- **In prophylaxis of haemorrhage**: Platelet count of <10 × 10^9/L coagulation disorders, petechiae, ecchymosis.
- **Prior to surgical or invasive procedures**, with platelet count of <50 × 10^9 L.
- **In case of microvascular bleeding without thrombocytopenia**, when impairment of platelet function is confirmed by laboratory tests. Platelets are transfused if this impairment cannot be treated by other ways (e.g. in case of congenital platelet disorders).
- Performing epidural anaesthesia or analgesia, with platelet count of <100 × 10^9/L.
- **In case of normal vaginal delivery,** thrombocytopenia of <50 × 10^9/L is safe without need for prophylactic platelet transfusion.

- Platelets should not be transfused (except the cases of life-threatening haemorrhage) under these circumstances: Auto-immune thrombocytopenia, thrombotic thrombocytopenic purpura, heparin-induced thrombocytopenia, post-trans-fusion purpura.

Following are the AABB guidelines for platelet transfusion[20]

Recommendation 1: The AABB recommends that platelets should be transfused prophylactically to reduce the risk for spontaneous bleeding in hospitalized adult patients with therapy induced hypoproliferative thrombocytopenia. **The AABB recommends transfusing hospitalized adult patients with a platelet count of 10×10^9 cells/L or less to reduce the risk for spontaneous bleeding.** The AABB recommends trans-fusing up to a single apheresis unit or equivalent. Greater doses are not more effective, and lower doses equal to one half of a standard apheresis unit are equally effective. (Grade: Strong recommendation; moderate-quality evidence)

Recommendation 2: The AABB suggests **prophylactic platelet transfusion for patients having elective central venous catheter placement with a platelet count less than 20×10^9 cells/L.** (Grade: Weak recommendation; low-quality evidence).

Recommendation 3: The AABB suggests **prophylactic platelet transfusion for patients having elective diagnostic lumbar puncture with a platelet count less than 50×10^9 cells/L.** (Grade: Weak recommendation; very low-quality evidence).

Recommendation 4: The AABB suggests **prophylactic platelet transfusion for patients having major elective non-neuraxial surgery with a platelet count less than 50×10^9 cells/L.** (Grade: Weak recommendation; very low-quality evidence).

Recommendation 5: The AABB recommends against routine prophylactic platelet transfusion for patients who are non-thrombocytopenic and have cardiac surgery with cardiopulmo-nary bypass. The AABB suggests platelet transfusion for patients having bypass who exhibit perioperative bleeding with thrombocytopenia and/or evidence of platelet dysfunction. (Grade: Weak recommendation; very low-quality evidence).

Recommendation 6: The AABB cannot recommend for or against platelet transfusion for patients receiving antiplatelet therapy who have intracranial haemorrhage (traumatic or spontaneous). (Grade: Uncertain recommendation; very-low-quality evidence).

An usual dose of platelets is 1 unit/10 kg or 1 therapeutic dose (consisting of 4–6 units of RDP), or 1 pack of apheresed platelets (SDP).

One unit of platelet concentrate (RDP) has on average 5.5–7.5 × 10^{10} of platelets.

Conventionally 5–10 × 10^9 of platelet increment per RDP is accepted after one hour of transfusion.

One unit of apheresed platelets has approximately **3.5–4 × 10^{11}** platelets and increases recipient's platelet count for 30–40 × 10^9/L.

Transfused platelets should raise the platelet count of recipients who have not been immunized or factors that reduce platelet survival.

The formula for calculating the corrected count increment is:

$$\frac{\text{Observed increment per } \mu l \times \text{Body surface area (m}^2)}{\text{Number of platelets given } (10^{11})}$$

Calculation of body surface area: Mosteller's formula

$$\sqrt{\frac{\text{Ht in cm} \times \text{Weight in kg}}{3600}}$$

After platelet transfusion, the therapeutic effect is evaluated after 60 minutes (1 hr), and again at 20–24 hours. Clinical studies have showed that the best time to evaluate the effectiveness of platelet transfusion is after 1 hour.

Failure to see the expected increment of platelets is mainly because of anti-platelet antibodies or splenomegaly (1 hour CCI reduced) or else due to decreased survival of the platelets as in sepsis, infections, DIC (24 hours CCI reduced).

From CCI, effective dose (ED) of platelets can be calculated.

$$ED = \frac{\text{Desired platelet increment} \times \text{Body surface area}}{\text{Expected CCI}}$$

Post-platelet recovery (PPR): This is the percentage of platelets (platelet increment) circulating in the blood after platelet transfusion. Usually 2/3rd of the platelets remain in circulation, if no splenomegaly or any other pathology of platelets exist. PPR of less than 20% suggests platelet refractoriness.

This is calculated by the following formula:

$$\frac{\text{Platelet increment per } \mu l \times \text{Estimated blood volume} \times 100}{\text{Number of platelet transfused } (10^{11})}$$

Transfusion of Fresh Frozen Plasma (FFP)

- **Fresh frozen plasma** is transfused, if in case of haemorrhage, the prothrombin time or activated partial thromboplastin time is prolonged for 1.5 times. If there is no haemorrhage, FFP should not be used for correction of hypovolemia or normalizing coagulation parameters. A recommended initial dose of FFP is **10–15 mL/kg** (average 3–4 units for a 70 kg adult patient); however, some repeated doses might be needed later on, after evaluation of therapeutic effect on bleeding.
- FFP can be stored for a year at –20°C. **FFP must be ABO compatible with the recipient's red blood cells.**
- FFP has been used as an exogenous source of proteins, especially albumin, immunoglobulins, coagulation factors and certain protease inhibitors.

Indications

- Coagulopathy and bleeding of different origin.
- Bleeding in case of disseminated intravascular coagulation (DIC).
- Thrombotic thrombocytopenic purpura.
- Congenital or acquired deficiency of different coagulation factors, when there is no possibility to get a certain factor concentrates (e.g. V or XI).
- Deficiency of specific plasma proteins (e.g. antithrombin III).
- Bleeding due to warfarin therapy.
- FFP should not be used when a coagulopathy can be corrected with vitamin K.

Transfusion of Cryoprecipitate

Indications

- Factor VIII deficiency.
- Haemorrhage due to hypofibrinogenemia or dysfibrinogenemia.
- DIC syndrome.
- von Willebrand's disease.
- Haemorrhage due to factor XIII deficiency.

Treating hypofibrinogenemia and transfusing cryoprecipitate of 1–2 units/10 kg increases plasma fibrinogen concentration for approximately 500 mg/L. Fibrinogen in plasma of 1 g/L is sufficient to maintain hemostasis.

Therapeutic Plasmapheresis or Plasma Exchange (TPE)

TPE is defined as removal of pathological plasma component and replacement of lost plasma with normal plasma, crystalloids and colloids. Generally exchange is limited to 40 mL/kg body weight (for 40 kg person 1600 mL) and lost plasma is replaced by crystalloids and colloids. Indications of TPE is given below.

Indications for Plasmapheresis

Goodpasture's syndrome (anti-GBM disease)

Myasthenia gravis crisis

Thrombotic thrombocytopenic purpura

Chronic inflammatory demyelinating polyneuropathy

Hemolytic uremic syndrome

Eaton-Lambert myasthenic syndrome

Cryoglobulinemia

Post-transfusion purpura

Hyperviscosity syndrome

Refsum's disease

Myeloma cast nephropathy

Cutaneous lymphoma (photopheresis)

Acute demyelinating polyneuropathy (Guillain-Barré)

HIV-related syndromes (polyneuropathy, hyperviscosity, TTP)

Homozygous familial hypercholesterolemia

Bullous pemphigoid

Rapidly progressive glomerulonephritis (without anti-GBM)

Pemphigus vulgaris

Paraproteinemic peripheral neuropathy

Immune thrombocytopenia

Systemic vasculitis associated with ANCA

Hemolytic disease of the newborn

ABO-incompatible marrow transplant

Bullous pemphigoid

SLE (particularly in SLE cerebritis)

Blood and Blood Component Transfusion in Obstetrics

- The **blood volume is markedly raised in pregnancy** due to the increased vascularity of the enlarging uterus with interposition of the utero-placental circulation. The rise is progressive and consistent. All the constituents are affected with increased blood volume. **The blood volume starts increasing from the 6th week, expands rapidly thereafter to maximum 40–50% above the non-pregnant level at 30–32 weeks. The level remains almost static till term.**
- **Plasma volume:** During pregnancy the **plasma volume is increased to the extent of 30–40%.** Total plasma volume increases to the extent of **1.25 litres.** This increase is greater in multigravida, multiple pregnancies and with large baby.
- The red cell volume is increased to the extent **of 20–30%.** The total increase in red cell volume is **350 mL.** The reticulocyte count increases by 2%. Erythropoietin level is raised.
- **There is disproportionate increase in plasma volume as compared to RBC volume which produces a state of hemo-dilution during pregnancy.**

TABLE 14.1: To show principle blood changes during pregnancy				
	Non-pregnant near term	Pregnancy increase	Total	% increase
Blood volume (mL)	4000 mL	5500 mL	1500 mL	30–40
Plasma volume (mL)	2500 mL	3750 mL	1250 mL	40–50
Red cell volume	1400 mL	1750 mL	350 mL	20–30
Haemoglobin (gm %)				
Haematocrit	38%	32%		18–20

- One woman dies from obstetric haemorrhage every minute.

The blood transfusions in pregnancy should be considered in the following instances:
- Acute blood loss of any amount with clinical evidence of inadequate oxygen carrying capacity or unstable vital signs.
- Symptomatic anaemia regardless of haemoglobin level even if no bleeding.

- Haemoglobin less than 7 gm, not amenable to other timely therapies, antenatally, intrapartum or immediately post-partum.
- Those receiving general anaesthesia, if the pre-operative haemoglobin is below 7 gm/dL.
- Caesarean section with haemoglobin less than 10 gm%.

Antepartum haemorrhage: Placenta previa and abruptio placenta are the two important causes of antepartum haemorrhage.

- Whenever the diagnosis of concealed variety of abruption has been made clinically, at least one litre of blood transfusion should be minimum to replenish the concealed blood loss irrespective of patient's general condition.

Peripartum/postpartum haemorrhage: Major obstetric haemorrhage can be peripartum and postpartum period. At term the blood flow to placenta is approximately 700 mL/minute. The patient's entire blood volume can be lost in 5–10 minutes. Unless the myometrium contracts on the placental site, blood loss will continue, even after the third stage of labour is complete.

- It is essential to monitor and investigate a patient with an obstetric haemorrhage, even in the absence of shock.
- Blood transfusion helps by **preventing ischemic renal damage by maintaining blood pressure**, prevents blood coagulation disorders and ensures patient to be in better form to withstand postpartum haemorrhage (PPH).
- Best indication to adequate blood replenishment rests on use of CVP which should be maintained at about 10 mm of H_2O.
- To maintain adequate organ perfusion, it is important to keep a haematocrit of 30%, urinary output of at least 30 mL/hr with IV fluids and blood.

Estimation of blood loss: Visual inspection is notoriously inaccurate. In obstetrics, part or all the haemorrhage may be concealed. It is important to realize that in a situation of acute blood loss **the immediate haematocrit may not reflect actual blood loss. After the loss of 1000 mL, the haematocrit typically** falls only 3 volume percent in the first hour. During the episode of acute significant haemorrhage, the initial haematocrit is always the highest.

ABO and Rh group with red cell antibody screening has to be carried out for a pregnant woman during her first visit to a doctor and at the 28th week of gestation. Another type of blood testing is cross-matching. It is performed to determine the compatibility of the donated blood with its intended recipient.

Crossmatching of blood should be requested under the following circumstances:

- Major antepartum, intrapartum and postpartum haemorrhage
- Placenta previa
- Severe pre-eclampsia or eclampsia
- Significant coagulation disorders
- Anaemia (when Hb <10 g/dL) prior to cesarean section
- Before an operation, when there are some significant obstetric abnormalities (uterine fibroids, previous classical caesarean section, previous placenta accreta)

Some of principles to be observed are as follows:

- For emergency cases, obstetric units should always reserve group 'O' Rh D negative, Kell-negative blood.
- In the absence of acute blood loss, ante-natal and post-natal patients should only be transfused when reduction of haemoglobin is associated with significant symptoms of anaemia.

Blood components used for transfusion in women of reproductive age must be Kell-negative in order to avoid alloimmunisation and subsequent haemolytic disease of the newborn (unless it is known that a woman is Kell-positive).

- If anti-K antibodies are found during pregnancy, they most likely have appeared due to previous transfusion, so this should be kept in mind concerning future red cell transfusions.
- It is recommended to use CMV-seronegative or leuco-depleted blood components (since it is thought that using leucocyte filters significantly reduces the risk of transmitting CMV).

However, in emergency circumstances, the transfusion should not be delayed if there are no CMV-seronegative blood components available.

Some precautionary measures by the treating obstetrician during pregnancy and delivery:

1. Clinician to care to maximize Hb at delivery
2. To minimize blood loss
3. Appropriate use of blood
4. Women with high risk pregnancy, to deliver at hospital with all facilities and intensive care
5. Use of tranexamic acid
6. Use of recombinant VIIa factor
7. Check-up at 28 weeks of pregnancy
8. If placenta previa keep 2 units of blood ready
9. Every week crossmatch and keep the units reserved.

RCOG Guidelines in Obstetrics[21]

1. If Hb level is less than 10.5 gm/dL in antenatal period, consider hematenic deficiency, once haemoglobinopathies have been excluded. **Oral iron should be preferred first line of treatment** for iron deficiency. **Parenteral iron is indicated when oral iron is not tolerated**, absorbed or patient compliance is in doubt. For parenteral therapy iron sucrose is given in multiple doses, whereas **iron dextran** may be given as single total dose infusion.

   Anaemia not due to iron deficiency should be managed by the blood transfusionist in close conjunction with haematologist.

   Transfusion almost always indicated when Hb is less than 6 gm/dL.

2. In pregnancy, pre-autologous deposit is not recommended.
3. Blood counts and coagulation screen are performed before giving FFP, cryoprecipitate and platelets.
4. Platelets should not fall below 50×10^9 in acute bleeding.

Neonatal Transfusion

- The total **blood volume of neonates is small**, although the volume is **higher per kg of body weight than that of older** children or adults (85 mL/kg for full-term and 100 to 105 mL/kg for pre-term).

- In neonates, a dose of 15 mL/kg of packed red blood cells will increase the haemoglobin by approximately 3 g/dL and 5 mL/kg of packed red blood cells will increase Hb by 1 gm%.
- Avoid using blood donated by blood relatives to transfuse neonates.
- Blood transfusion in pre-term infants is often given for the anaemia of prematurity (associated with delayed renal production of erythropoietin due to decreased sensitivity to lower haematocrit levels). This commonly develops in neonates **after 2 weeks** of life. Neonates, especially pre-term, may require multiple transfusions.
- Blood component therapy is a very common intervention practiced in newborns; nearly 85% of extremely low birth weight (ELBW) babies get transfusions during their hospital stay.
- **Indications of packed red blood cells (PRBCs) for transfusion in neonatal practice:** PRBCs are the most commonly used blood product in neonatal transfusions. Indications for transfusion of PRBCs are mainly resolution of symptomatic anaemia and for improvement of tissue oxygenation. Tissue oxygenation depends on cardiac output, oxygen saturation and haemoglobin concentration. Once cardiac output and oxygen saturation are optimal, tissue oxygenation can only be improved by increasing the haemoglobin level.

Canadian Paediatric Society recommends[22] following guidelines for red blood cell transfusion in newborns:

1. Group O Rh-negative blood may be used in the emergency transfusion of newborns. Otherwise, either group O Rh-compatible or group-specific Rh-compatible blood must be used. Starting at four months postnatal age, crossmatching of donor blood is required (strong recommendation).

2. In cases of massive haemorrhage, for which a large volume of blood may be required, care should be taken to avoid hyperkalemia and dilution of coagulation factors, using combined replacement with fresh blood or frozen plasma, as necessary (strong recommendation).

3. 'Top-up' transfusions should be used to maintain haemo-globin levels >7.5 gm/dL in convalescent preterm infants (moderate recommendation).
4. For infants in the first and second week of life, minimum haemoglobin levels of 10 gm/dL and 8.5 gm/dL, respectively, are recommended (weak recommendation).
5. Infants needing respiratory support may require transfusion at higher haemoglobin thresholds (weak recommendation).
6. Infants with cyanotic heart disease or similar haemodynamic disorders may require transfusion at higher haemoglobin thresholds (weak recommendation).
7. Transfusions should not be used to improve weight gain or to address apnea of prematurity when haemoglobin levels are already in excess of recommended levels for maintenance (weak recommendation).

The guidelines for transfusion of PRBC vary according to age, level of sickness and haematocrit.

TABLE 14.2: Guidelines for packed red blood cells (PRBCs) transfusion thresholds for preterm neonates[23]	
Less than 28 days of age	1. Assisted ventilation with FiO_2 more than 0.3: Hb 12.0 gm/dL or PCV less than 40%
	2. Assisted ventilation with FiO_2 less than 0.3: Hb 11.0 g/dL or PCV less than 35%
	3. CPAP: Hb less than 10 gm/dL or PCV less than 30%
More than 28	1. Assisted ventilation: Hb less than 10 gm/dL or days of age PCV less than 30%
	2. CPAP: Hb less than 8 gm/dL or PCV less than 25%
Any age, breathing spontaneously	1. On FiO_2 more than 0.21: Hb less than 8 gm/dL or PCV less than 25%
	2. On room air: Hb less than 7 gm/dL or PCV less than 20%

Red cells collected in CPDA-1 are kept as packed RBCs. CPDA-1 packed RBCs have a haematocrit of approximately 75% and a shelf life of 35 days. An infusion **of 10 mL/kg of CPDA-1 packed RBCs** would be expected to raise the patient's haematocrit by **9% to 10**%.

CMV reduced RBCs are used to reduce the risk of transmitting CMV, which may be a cause of considerable concern in newborns. **CMV reduction** can be achieved by either **leukoreduction** of blood components, or by pre-selecting **donors who are CMV negative**. Providing CMV reduced blood is important in preterm infants, as preterm neonates can have severe form of CMV infection than term newborns.

Practical issues

1. **Amount of transfusion to be given:** It has been seen that transfusion with PRBCs at a dose of **20 mL/kg** is well tolerated and results in an overall decrease in number of transfusions compared to transfusions done at **10 mL/ kg**. There is also a higher rise in haemoglobin with a higher dose of PRBCs.

2. **Properties of RBC products used in neonatal transfusion:** **RBCs** should be freshly prepared and **should not be more than 7 days old**. This translates into a high 2, 3-DPG concentration and higher tissue extraction of oxygen. Other concerns with **old RBCs are: Hyperkalemia, and a reduced RBC life span**. In small and sick neonates, where it is anticipated that blood component therapy may be needed more than once, it may help to have aliquots from a single donor given as sequential transfusions. **This is done practically by reserving a bag of fresh PRBCs for up to 7 days for a newborn and withdrawing small aliquots required repeatedly from that bag under laminar flow using a sterile connecting device**, into a fresh blood bag. The PRBC bag is immediately resealed under the laminar flow, and can be re-used for withdrawing similar small quantities of blood for up to 7 days.

3. The infant's Hb concentration at birth tends to be approximately 16.5 gm/dL and increases to 18.4 gm/dL within 24 hours at birth. During first 3 months of life all infants will have a normal or physiological decrease in their Hb down to approximately to 11.5 gm/dL. This decrease is greater in pre-term infants. By 12 years of age, the Hb levels will be as those of adults.[24]

4. At birth until six months of age, the concentration of vitamin K dependent coagulation factors (factors II, VII, IX and X) and vitamin K dependent inhibitors of coagulation (protein C and S) are lower than adult levels. By age of 6 months they will reach the levels approximately as that of adults.[24]

Choosing the blood group for neonatal transfusion:

1. It is preferable to take samples from both, mother and the newborn, for initial testing prior to transfusion. **Mother's sample should be tested for blood group and for any atypical red cell antibodies**.

2. ABO compatibility is essential while transfusing PRBCs. Though **ABO antigens may be expressed** only weakly on neonatal erythrocytes, neonate's serum may contain transplacentally acquired maternal IgG anti-A and/or anti-B.

3. **Blood should be of newborn's ABO and Rh group**. It should be compatible with ABO or red cell antibodies present in the maternal serum.

4. In **exchange transfusions** for haemolytic disease of newborn, **blood transfused should be compatible with mother's serum. If the mother's and the baby's blood groups are the same, use Rh negative blood of baby's ABO group. In case mother's and baby's blood group is not compatible, use group O and Rh negative** blood for exchange transfusion. For exchange transfusion, red cells should be less than 5 days old, sickle screen negative, collected in CPD anticoagulant and gamma irradiated.

Volume and rate of transfusion:

a. Volume of packed RBCs = Blood volume (mL/kg) × (desired minus actual haematocrit)/haematocrit of transfused RBC.

b. Rate of infusion should be less than 10 mL/kg/hour in the absence of cardiac failure.

c. Rate should not be more than 2 mL/kg/hour in the presence of cardiac failure.

d. If more volume is to be transfused, it should be done in smaller aliquots.

Expected response: Each transfusion of 9 mL/kg of body weight should increase haemoglobin level by 3 g/dL. Meticulous monitoring of input, output and vital signs are mandatory during blood transfusion.

Neonatal Platelet Transfusion[25–29]

1. For a stable neonate <20,000 platelets/cmm
2. If unstable neonate <30,000 platelets/cmm
3. With active bleeding <50,000 platelets/cmm

Practical issues for platelet transfusion in neonates

1. Platelets should **never be filtered through a micropore blood filter before transfusion**, as it will considerably decrease the number of platelets.
2. **Rh-negative infants** should receive platelets from **Rh-negative donors** to prevent Rh sensitization from the contaminating red blood cells.
    1. The usual recommended dose of platelets for neonates is **1 unit of platelet per 10 kg body weight,** which amounts to **5 mL/kg.** The predicted rise in platelet count from a 5 mL/kg dose would be **20 to 60,000/cubic mm**. Doses of up to 10–20 mL/kg may be used in case of severe thrombocytopenia.
    2. Platelet count should not fall below 50,000/cmm in preterm neonates who exhibit active bleeding or at a great risk of bleeding by an invasive procedure.[25–29]
    3. In the selection of platelets units for transfusion, it is desirable that the infant and the platelet donor to be of the same ABO blood group.
    4. Repeated transfusions of O group platelets to A or B recipients should be minimized in view of the anti-A and anti-B antibodies causing lysis of the red cells.[25–29]

Following are to be kept in mind while transfusing the neonate:

- **Infectious complications:** In India, it is mandatory to test every unit of blood collected for hepatitis B, hepatitis C, HIV/AIDS, syphilis and malaria. However, transfusion transmitted infections are still a considerable risk, because of the relative insensitivity of screening tests, and several other organisms besides those tested for, which may be transmitted through blood.

- **Non-infectious complications:** These can be immune mediated and non-immune mediated reactions, or can classified as acute and delayed complications.

- **Immune mediated haemolysis:** Acute haemolytic transfusion reactions are common causes of transfusion related fatality in adult patients, but these are rare in neonates. Newborns do not have red blood cell (RBC) antibodies; all antibodies present are maternal in origin.

- Newborns must be screened for maternal RBC antibodies, including ABO antibodies if non-O blood group transfusion to be given as the first transfusion.

- If the initial results are negative, no further testing is needed for the initial few post-natal months. Infants are at a **higher risk of passive immune haemolysis from infusion of ABO incompatible plasma present in PRBCs or platelet concentrates.** Smaller quantities of ABO-incompatible plasma (less than 5 mL/kg) are generally well tolerated. **Newborns do not manifest the usual symptoms of haemolysis that are observed in older patients,** such as fever, hypotension, and flank pain. An acute haemolytic event may be present as increased pallor, presence of plasma free haemoglobin, haemoglobinuria, increased serum potassium levels, and acidosis. Results of the direct antiglobulin (Coombs') test may confirm the presence of an antibody on the RBC surface. Treatment is mainly supportive and involves maintenance of blood pressure and kidney perfusion with intravenous saline bolus of 10 to 20 mL/kg along with forced diuresis with furosemide. Enforcing strict guidelines for patient identification and issue of blood; and minimizing human error is essential in preventing immune mediated haemolysis.

- **Fluid overload:** Neonates are at increased risk of fluid overload from transfusion because the volume of the blood component issued may exceed the volume that may be transfused safely into neonates. Care should be taken to ensure that, in the absence of blood loss, **volumes infused**

do not exceed 10 to 20 mL/kg. There is no role for routine use of furosemide while transfusing newborns.

- **Metabolic complications:** These complications occur with large volume of transfusions like exchange transfusions.
  a. **Hyperkalemia: In stored blood, potassium levels tend to be high**. It has been seen that after storage for around 42 days, potassium levels may reach 50 mEq/L in a RBC unit. Though small volume transfusions do not have much risk of metabolic disturbances, large volume transfusions may lead to hyperkalemia. **Washing PRBCs before reconstituting with FFP before exchange transfusion helps in preventing this complication**.
  b. **Hypoglycemia: Blood stored in CPD blood has a high content of glucose leading to a rebound rise in insulin release, 1–2 hours after transfusion. This may lead to hypoglycaemia** and routine monitoring is necessary, particularly after exchange transfusion, after 2 and 6 hours, to ensure that this complication does not occur.
  c. **Acid–base derangements:** Metabolism of citrate in CPD leads to late metabolic alkalosis. Metabolic acidosis is an immediate complication occurring in sick babies who cannot metabolize citrate.
  d. **Hypocalcemia and hypomagnesemia:** These are caused by binding of these ions by citrate present in CPD blood.
- **Transfusion associated graft-versus-host disease (TA-GvHD):** Newborns are at risk for TA-GvHD, if they have received intrauterine transfusions or exchange transfusions. Unchecked donor T cell proliferation is the cause of TA-GvHD, and it can be effectively prevented by leuco-reduction and irradiation of the transfused blood.

Blood and Blood Component Transfusion in Paediatric Patients

- Blood transfusions are life saving in modern intensive care of premature neonates, children with cancer, children with haemolytic anaemias, coagulation disorders and children requiring transplants. The principles of transfusion in children and adolescents are similar to those of adults, but infant has special needs.

- Transfusions are not without any risks and are to given only when true benefits are likely.
- **A clear indication of transfusion must exist;** otherwise, the child may be unnecessarily subjected to the risk of transfusion associated problems.
- Components should not be unpacked until just before transfusion. An informed consent from parents after explaining the procedure and expected outcome must be taken. The blood can be warmed in a water bath which is thermostatically controlled, to ensure that the temperature of the water bath does not exceed 42°C. Adjust flow rate as outlined and never transfuse beyond 4 hours. Never inject any medication into transfusion line.

Guidelines for Transfusion of RBCs in Full-term Infant under 4 Months of Age[25–29]

Hb less than 7 gm/dL with low reticulocyte count and with symptoms of anaemia Hb less than 10 gm/dL in an infant:

- On <35% hood O_2
- On O_2 by nasal canula
- On ventilation with mean airway pressure of <6 cm of H_2O
- With significant tachycardia and tachypnea
- With significant apnea and bradycardia

Hb less than 12 gm/dL in an infant:

- On >35% hood O_2
- On continuous ventilation with mean airway pressure of 6–8 cm of H_2O

Hb of 15 gm/dL in an infant:

- On ECMO
- With congenital cyanotic heart disease

For more than 4 months of age[25–29]

1. Acute blood loss more than 15% of total blood volume
2. Hb less than 7 gm/dL with symptomatic anaemia
3. Significant pre-operative anaemia when corrective therapy is not available
4. Hb less than 13 gm/dL on ECMO

5. Chronic transfusion programs for disorders of RBC production.

Guidelines for Platelet Transfusion in Children

1. **5–10,000 platelets/cmm** with **failure of platelet production.**
2. **<30,000 platelets/cmm** in a neonate with **failure of platelet production.**
3. **<50,000 platelets/cmm** in premature neonate with active bleeding and in cases of invasive procedures.
4. <1,00,000 platelets/cmm in a sick premature with active bleeding and invasive procedures.

Autologous Blood Transfusion

Introduction

Autologous blood transfusion is the collection of blood from a person and re-transfusion back to the same person when required. This is in contrast to allogenic blood transfusion, where blood from unrelated/unknown donors is transfused to the recipient. The main aim for the use of autologous blood transfusion is to reduce the risk of transmission of infection.

In 1937, Fantus proposed autologous donation (pre-operative).

Methods of Autologous Blood Transfusion[30,31]

There are three methods of autologous transfusion.

- **Cell salvage:** Blood is collected from suction, surgical drains, or both and re-transfused back to the patient after filtration or washing.
- **Pre-operative autologous donation (PAD):** Blood is collected in advance before an elective procedure, stored in the blood bank and transfused back to the patient when required.
- **Acute normovolaemic haemodilution (ANH):** Blood is collected immediately prior to surgery and blood volume is restored by crystalloids or colloids. The blood is then re-transfused towards the end of surgery once haemostasis is achieved.

Advantages

1. In patients with rare blood groups beneficial.
2. In autoimmune haemolytic anaemia, when compatible blood is not available.

3. To reduce transfusion of infections.
4. Cell salvage can be utilized when no alternative is available to save the life.

Disadvantages: The use of autologous blood transfusion is not without risk and complications. This adds to increased cost and therefore should only be considered in certain situations. Strict protocols and guidelines must be in place to ensure patient safety.

Cell Salvage

This technique can be performed intra-operatively, post-operatively or by both ways. The process involves collection of shed blood from the surgical field. The salvaged blood is then either filtered or washed and processed prior to re-transfusion back to the patient in the immediate postoperative period.

Advantages: Red blood cells which would have been lost are scavenged and re-infused. The technique provides a supply of red blood cells in proportion to the losses. This provides a means of reducing the requirement of allogenic blood transfusion.

Disadvantages: Intraoperative cell salvage requires complex specialized instrument and a high level of training for the operator. The process is complex and can result in serious complications.

Preoperative Autologous Donation (PAD)

- This process commences up to 5 weeks prior to surgery (defined by the limit of conventional blood storage techniques) allowing the collection of up to 4–6 units of blood. Oral or IV iron supplementation (for faster increase in haemoglobin) may be required to maintain erythropoiesis.
- The last donation should take place at least 48–72 hours before the surgery to allow equilibration of blood volume.
- The blood is collected into blood bags and stored in the blood bank in a conventional manner. It should be clearly labeled to identify it from allogenic units.

- At the time of surgery, the pre-donated blood is issued from the blood bank as required in the conventional manner.

Criteria for Autologous Donation

- **Hb:** 11 gm/dL or haematocrit 33% or higher.
- **Age:** No upper or lower limit.
- **Weight:** Blood drawn is adjusted using the formula. Anticoagulant added also needs to be adjusted.
- **Frequency of donation:** Not less than every 3 days and not less than 72 hours before surgery.

In certain occasions **"Frog Leap"** technique can be used to collect autologous blood which needs close observation by the physician and blood bank staff. With this procedure on day 36, about 6 units of blood can be kept ready before surgery.

Phlebotomy day	Units drawn	Units re-infused	Number of units available
Day 1	1	None	1
Day 8	2	1	2
Day 15	4	2	3
Day 22	6	3	4
After 28 days	8	4	5
Day 36	10	5	6

Advantages

- The technique provides up to 4–6 units of blood, which will cover many elective operations and eliminate the need of blood from other donors. The risks of viral transmission and immunologically mediated haemolytic, febrile or allergic reaction are virtually eliminated provided the patient only receives autologous blood. Immune-modulation seen after allogenic transfusion does not occur.

- Autologous blood transfusion, when used appropriately, can provide a safe alternative to allogenic blood transfusion. However, there will always be a need for allogenic blood (even patients who have autologous blood, may need further transfusion with allogenic units).

Disadvantages

- The system requires a great deal of logistic planning well ahead of surgery. This may be a particular problem where surgery is re-scheduled at short notice. Pre-donated blood must be clearly labeled in the blood bank and the risk of clerical or human error remains. Up to 50% of pre-donated blood is unused; this wastage together with costs of administering PAD results in higher cost per unit of blood in comparison with allogenic blood.

Acute Normovolaemic Haemodilution (ANH)

- The blood collected just prior to surgery is re-transfused after surgery. This procedure can replace allogenic blood transfusion, increase the level of anaemia tolerance and adaptation to volume and red cell loss. ANH in cardiac surgery can reduce blood viscosity during hypothermia. Not only in adults, elderly, neonates and children but also in all types of surgeries like orthopaedic, gynaecological, urological and vascular surgeries, ANH can be beneficial.

- Relative contraindications are in patient of unstable angina pectoris, severe coronary artery stenosis, CCF, COPD, etc. Blood collection is usually done after induction of anaesthesia and before surgical blood loss occurs. The blood must be labeled with patients' name, identification no. and time of withdrawal. It is stored at room temperature in the operation room and should be infused at the end of the surgery or infuse earlier if signs of hypoxia occur. The blood withdrawn is replaced by crystalloids and colloids. Thus, there is maintenance of normovolaemia.

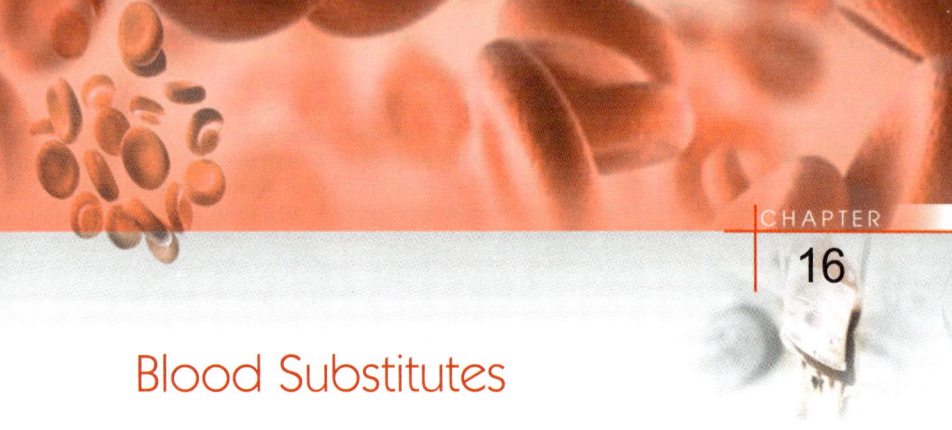

Blood Substitutes

Developing a safe blood substitute has been a goal of medical researchers for decades, promoted by the traumas of both World Wars, as well as more recent wars in Asia and the Middle East. Further efforts for development of blood substitutes are mainly due to blood-borne infections, especially hepatitis B and C, and HIV.

The two major classes of oxygen-carrying blood substitutes[2] studied are the haemoglobin-based oxygen carriers and perfluorocarbon emulsions.

Haemoglobin-Based Oxygen Carriers (HBOCs)

HBOCs are solutions that contain haemoglobin from purified. human, animal, or recombinant sources. HBOCs prepared from various sources have been investigated; one such product is available for veterinary use (bovine derived), and another for human use in South Africa (bovine derived). While no HBOC is anticipated to replace allogenic blood, a safe HBOC would facilitate haemodynamic stabilization until blood is available, and do so without concern for infectious agent transmission or transfusion reactions. HBOCs benefit when blood is in short supply or unavailable.

Haemoglobin provides oxygen-carrying capacity, transportation, and the modulation of other biochemical processes. The haemoglobin normally contained in red blood cells (RBCs) is a tetramer of two alpha and two beta polypeptide chains that are bound to a central protoporphyrin ring. When the natural haemoglobin molecule escapes RBCs, it rapidly dissociates into dimers composed of an alpha and a beta subunit that does not transport oxygen well. Thus, it is only inside RBCs that the iron-containing protoporphyrin ring (heme group) binds one oxygen molecule causing conformational changes that further increases the affinity of haemoglobin for added oxygen. This variable affinity for oxygen is the basis of the oxygen-haemoglobin dissociation curve, and alterations in oxygen delivery are modulated by temperature, pH changes, or 2,3-diphosphoglycerate.

Haemoglobin solutions have a lower P50 (higher affinity) of 12–14 mm Hg compared with normal values for RBCs of ~27 mm Hg, which compromises the liberation of oxygen to the periphery. For therapeutic use, purified haemoglobins have undergone multiple chemical modifications, including cross-linking, conjugation and polymerization to other compounds to change their physiochemical characteristics.

Polymerised haemoglobin (PolyHb), is haemoglobin product cross-linked and polymerized with glutaraldehyde and o-raffinose/pyridoxol molecules to increase its ability to deliver oxygen and increase its duration of action in circulation. The limited duration of efficacy is due to increased clearance of free haemoglobin in circulation, and auto-oxidation to methaemoglobin. PolyHb is still in trial phase.

Diaspirin, a product produced by US Army, is a cross-linked haemoglobin (DCLHb). The cross-linking agent is bis (dibromosalicyl) fumarate (DBBF). This has shelf life of 9 months, however, has side effects like intense vasoconstriction, reduced cardiac output and increased vascular resistance. Because of the adverse effects the production has been discontinued.

Although HBOCs cannot replace allogeneic red blood cells completely, they may be used in special circumstances, including instances of life-threatening haemorrhage, or when allogeneic RBCs are not available. However, defining the studies to allow these to be approved by regulatory agencies is exceedingly difficult. One of the major problems in using HBOCs in shock states is that free haemoglobin in solution avidly binds nitric oxide, and thus may impair regional auto-regulation of blood flow in major organ systems, causing vasoconstriction and hypoperfusion. In preclinical and animal models, free haemoglobin is an important mechanism responsible for organ injury.

Allogeneic RBCs and HBOCs are not equivalent; RBCs are more effective oxygen-carrying agents. Although studies demonstrate that HBOCs reduce allogeneic RBC transfusions in elective surgical procedures, several units are required to replace one unit of allogeneic blood. HBOCs have different side effects; most commonly related to nitric oxide scavenging, their side effect profile is a difficult problem. Given the widespread civilian availability of allogeneic RBCs and the appearance of excess mortality with HBOCs, many trials have been held, suspended, or abandoned. There is no current FDA approval for these agents.

Perfluorocarbon Emulsions (PFCs)

PFCs are a class of hydrocarbons produced by substitution of single hydrogen of each carbon atom of benzene ring with fluoride radical in the selected hydrocarbon base and have the following properties.

1. These are chemically inert molecules, clear and colorless liquids.
2. They can dissolve many gases including O_2 and CO_2 gases.
3. They carry these gases all over the body.
4. They are not miscible and need to be emulsified for intravenous administration.
5. Their ability to carry O_2 is directly proportion to their concentration in blood, importantly to the partial pressure of oxygen in blood.
6. These PFCs can flow in the microcirculation, can perfuse even the tiniest capillary and augment oxygen delivery, much more than what would be expected from an increase in oxygen content alone.
7. All the oxygen carried by these PFCs is in a dissolved state, resulting in a higher oxygen partial pressure, thus augmenting the driving pressure for diffusion of dissolved oxygen into the tissues.

PFCs have great value in treatment of myocardial infarction, thrombosis, atherosclerosis and vasculo-occlusive diseases carrying oxygen beyond the occluded area.

The first generation PFC is **Fluosol (Green Cross)** uses poloxamer type Pleuronic F-68 as an emulsifier. However, this emulsifier can produce anaphylaxis and complement activation. The second generation PFC is **Oxygent**, uses egg yolk phospholipids as an emulsifier which is well tolerated and also contains a stabilizer perflubrodec (Perfluorodecyl bromide-$C10F21Br$).

Recombinant Haemoglobin

This is cross-linked haemoglobin genetically produced in organisms like *E. coli* or saccharomyces cerevisae yeast. This also has adverse effects like vasoconstriction, GI distress, fever, chills and backache, hence trials have been discontinued.

Role of Nanotechnology

Nanotechnology can be used to develop artificial haemoglobin. Cross-linking haemoglobin into PolyHb of nano dimensional structure, artificial cells can be prepared in the form of lipid vesicles containing haemoglobin or haemoglobin containing biodegradable membrane. This technology is safe, does not cause complement activation or adverse effects, but still in trial phase.

Artificial RBCs

Development of synthetic haemoglobin and combining with functional enzymes similar to natural RBCs has been tried. These RBCs have short life and an attempt to prepare artificial RBCs is not successful.

Lipid Membrane Artificial Cells

Incorporation of polyethylene glycol (PEG) into lipid membrane of artificial RBCs has increased circulation half time of more than 30 hours. Biodegradable polymers, such as polylactic acid (PLA) for the microencapsulation of Hb, enzymes and other materials have been used in place of lipid membrane. Haemoglobin nanocapsule prepared with PLA can survive for longer time in circulation. Enzymes such as methaemoglobin reductase have been incorporated into the membrane. This membrane also allows ascorbic acid to pass inside the cell. These efforts are to prevent methaemoglobin formation and longer survival of the cells.

HLA Antigens and other Platelet and Leucocyte Antigens and their Role in Blood Transfusion

Antigens expressed on leucocytes and platelets

These include:
- HLA antigens
- Blood group antigens on other cells
- Other antigens

Role of HLA in Blood Banking

The **human leucocyte antigen (HLA)** system is the name of the major histocompatibility complex (MHC) in humans. The locus contains a large number of genes related to immune function.

HLA antigens are major histocompatibility complex (MHC) molecules and have the following functions and characteristics:
- The HLA system is highly polymorphic, there are many alleles of each MHC gene in the population.
- This complex contains 35–40 genes and is clustered on chromosome 6p21.3.
- MHC molecules have key roles in regulating T cell mediated immune response.
- Display peptide fragments of proteins for recognition by antigen-specific T cells.

HLA Antigens

- **Class I A, B and C antigens are expressed on all the cells except spermatozoa, trophoblastic cells and RBCs.** They are expressed on **platelets and leucocytes also**. On RBC membrane, these can be adsorbed from the plasma.

- Platelets possess mRNA encoding HLA class I molecule and are capable of synthesizing them.

The proteins encoded by certain genes are also known as *antigens*, the major HLA antigens are essential elements for immune function. HLA antigens corresponding to MHC class I (A, B, C) present peptides from inside the cell (including viral peptides, if present). These peptides are produced from digested proteins that are broken down in the proteosomes. In general, the peptides are small polymers about 9 amino acids in length. These antigens attract CD8 positive cytotoxic T cells that destroy them.

Class II antigens are on lymphocytes, monocytes, macrophages, activated T cells and Langerhan's cells.

HLA antigens corresponding to MHC class II (DP, DM, DOA, DOB, DQ and DR) present antigens from outside of the cell to T-lymphocytes. These particular antigens stimulate the multiplication of T-helper cells, which in turn stimulate antibody-producing B-cells to produce antibodies to that specific antigen. Self-antigens are suppressed by suppressor T-cells.

HLA Antibodies

HLA antibodies are typically not naturally occurring. They are formed as a result of an immunologic challenge of a foreign material containing non-self HLAs via blood transfusion, pregnancy (paternally-inherited antigens), or organ or tissue transplant.

The HLA system has important implications in transfusion therapy. Sensitization of recipients with consecutive formation of HLA antibodies and is the cause for thrombocytopenia and may cause febrile transfusion reactions.

Blood Group Antigens on Other Cells

- A, B antigens are present on lymphocytes and are detected by lymphocytotoxicity tests. Lewis antigens are acquired from plasma.
- A, B and H antigens are on platelets.

- Epidermal cells, cells of amniotic fluid, sinusoidal cells of spleen, spermatozoa, endothelial cells have A, B and H antigens.

Other Antigens

- Human neutrophil antigens (HNA)
- Platelet specific antigens

Human Neutrophil/Granulocyte Antigens (HNA)

- Neutrophil specific antigens like HNA1 (1a and 1b), HNA2 and SH are present on the neutrophils.
  Other antigens on neutrophils are HNA 2a, HNA 3a, HNA 4a and HNA 5a.
- Antibodies develop when the person lacks these antigens, antibodies to **HNA1-1a** and **1b** are often implicated.
  These are recognised by Fc portion of the IgG.
  Granulocyte specific antibodies (HNA-1a and 1b) **and HLA class I antibodies** are responsible for:
- Neonatal allo and isoimmune neutropenia
- Febrile non-haemolytic transfusion reactions
- Transfusion related acute lung injury (TRALI)
- Auto-immune neutropenia
  In platelet packs and RBC packs, the granulocytes release cytokines with storage, hence pre-storage leuco-reduction is preferred.

Alloimmunization

Leucocytes in blood products are the major stimulus for allo-immunization. The number of leucocytes in different blood is given below.

PRBCs: $2–5 \times 10^9$ WBCs.

Random platelets: $0.5–2.5 \times 10^8$ WBCs.

Leucoreduced: Less than 5.0×10^6 WBCs.

Neonatal alloimmune neutropenia is similar to haemolytic disease of newborn with following possibilities:
- Passively transmitted maternal antibodies.

- Mother's serum has potent IgG antibodies against granulocyte specific antigens.
- Usually 1st child is affected.

Neonatal Iso-immune Neutropenia

This develops in subjects in whom the glycoprotein is absent on the granulocytes due to deletion of the gene, may form strong antibodies.

Infants born to these mothers will suffer from iso-immune neutropenia.

Febrile Non-Haemolytic Transfusion Reactions (FNHTRs)

For details refer to transfusion reactions.

As a remedy for these reactions, leucocyte reduction is preferred.

Pre-storage leucocyte reduction is preferred with less than 5×10^6 leucocytes and 85% RBCs to be retained.

Leukofilters with
- Barrier filtration: Pore size smaller than WBCs.
- Cell adhesion are used.

Note: For details refer to transfusion reactions.

Transfusion Related Lung Injury (TRALI)

For details refer to transfusion reactions.

Transfusion-Associated Graft-Versus-Host Disease (TA-GVHD)

For details refer to transfusion reactions.

Tests done to detect antibodies:
- Granulocyte agglutination
- Immunofluroscence (IF)
- Chemiluminescence
- Monoclonal antibody specific immobilisation of granulocyte assays.

Granulocyte agglutination technique:
- Granulocyte suspension is prepared by dextran sedimentation followed by centrifugation on ficoll-hypaque.

- The RBCs are lysed with ammonium chloride or distilled water or WBCs are obtained by double density gradient centrifugation.
- Agglutination carried out on microplates.
- They are agglutinated by cross-linking of cells by IgM or IgG antibodies which adhere to Fc receptors on granulocytes.
- Granulocyte specific antibodies and HLA A, B and C antibodies can be detected. HLA A, B and C antibodies can be better detected with lymphotoxicity tests.

Platelet Antigens

HLA antibodies to HLA class I antigen after transfusion are the major cause of antibody mediated refractoriness to platelet transfusion, febrile transfusion reactions and occur in pregnancy.

Allo-antibodies to HLA class I antigen on platelets and antibodies to platelet specific antigens occur in neonatal alloimmune thrombocytopenia (NAT/NAIT), post-transfusion purpura (PTP), **passive alloimmune transfusion** (PAT) and transplantation associated purpura. **Anti-platelet specific antibodies** are detected in 8% of recipients of **multiple platelet transfusions.**

Post-transfusion Purpura

- Rare complication.
- Rapid onset of thrombocytopenia as a result of anamnestic production of platelet allo-antibodies.
- Usually occurs in multi-parous women who do not have the antigen.
- Multiple transfusion recipients.
- Allo-antibodies in the recipient clear the donor platelets.

Alloimmunisation to Platelet Specific Antigens

Post-transfusion purpura is a mystery of alloimmunisation.

- Sudden decrease in platelet counts 7–10 days post-transfusion.

• Recipient is negative for the platelet antigen (usually PLA1 or Br^a). Usually under diagnosed or diagnosed after severe bleed.

Mechanism

Majority of population is PLA1 positive and thus majority of donors are PLA1 positive. Pl-A1 is a soluble antigen. When Pl-A1 negative individuals receive PLA1 positive products, Pl-A1 antigens bind to PLA1 negative platelets. Pl-A1 is recognized as a foreign and antibodies are produced. Antibody binds to PLA1 antigen. Pl-A1 antigen is removed from circulation.

Errors and Discrepancies in ABO Typing

In the ABO system of blood groups, if an antibody is present in the serum, the reciprocal antigen will be absent from the red cell membrane and vice versa is true. When the cell grouping does not correlate with the serum grouping, there is said to be a discrepancy in ABO grouping.

Mistyping either a donor or recipient can lead to transfusion with ABO-incompatible blood. ABO antibodies can activate complement and result *in vivo* haemolysis. The clinical consequences of this *in vivo* destruction can be significant and may even result in death of the recipient.

Most errors being technical errors and clerical errors, other ABO discrepancies can be classified into 4 categories:
Category I: Weakly reacting or missing antigens
Category II: Weakly reacting or missing antibodies
Category III: Unexpected antigen reactions
Category IV: Unexpected antibody reactions

Technical errors and clerical errors
1. Incorrect labeling
2. Mix-up of samples
3. Poor quality/expired reagents/red cells
4. Contaminated reagents
5. Inappropriate storage temperature
6. Failure to add reagents
7. Failure to follow manufacturer's instructions
8. Missed observation by untrained staff

9. Equipment variables
10. Uncalibrated instruments
11. Contaminated glassware
12. Wrong entry of results
13. Transcription error
14. Computer entry error

Resolution: Re-check the label. Ask for new sample.

Check for red cell suspension or freshly prepare the red cell suspension. Check QC of reagents.

Check equipment.

Verify the patient data for previous blood group report and history of transfusion.

Category I: Weakly Reacting or Missing Antigens

ABO subgroups (subgroups of A or B): Rare subgroups of a like A2, Ax, Am, Ae, etc. have weak antigens. Sometimes associated with presence of Anti-A1 antibodies.

In forward grouping appears as O, but reverse grouping appears as A or B. A example is given below.

	Antibodies			Cells				
	Anti-A	Anti-B	Anti-AB	A1	A2	B	O	Auto
1 min spin	0	0	0	0	0	4+	0	0
RT 15 min	0	0	1+	0	0	4+	0	0
4°C 30 min	1+	0	2+	1+	0	4+	0	0

Note: Weak subgroup of A (A2), reaction can be enhanced by incubation at room temperature and at 4°C. Anti-A1 can be demonstrated in serum at 4°C. Antibody screen for O cells and auto control should be performed.

Resolution: Incubation at room temperature and 4°C will enhance the reactivity of antibodies. ABO antibodies at cold temperature of 4°C incubation can demonstrate weak reacting antigen.

ABO subgroups can be classified based on strength of agglutination with ABO antisera.

Pathologic causes: In acute leukemia there is weakened expression of A and B antigens.

Carcinoma of stomach and pancreas: There can be excess of soluble blood group substances in the plasma which may neutralize the anti-A and anti-B antibodies causing **a false negative** reaction.

Resolution: Washing removes blood specific substances. Only red cells will remain with washing which gives correct grouping.

	Antibodies			Cells			
	Anti-A	Anti-B	Anti-AB	A1	B	O	Auto
Unwashed RBCs	0	0	0	4+	0	0	0
Washed RBCs	0	4+	4+				

Note: With washed RBCs, it is B blood group.

Category II: Weakly Reacting or Missing Antibodies

Antibodies			Cells			
Anti-A	Anti-B	Anti-AB	A1 cells	B cells	O cells	Auto
0	0	0	0	0	0	0

Note: In the above example, with cell grouping it is O blood group, but reverse grouping no antibodies are detected with A1, B and O cells. Possible cause is—infant, elderly or pathological cause such as hypogammaglobulinemia. In such case check the age and diagnosis of the case.

Weakly reacting or missing antibodies are found in the following conditions.

- **Newborns:** Missing antibodies in reverse grouping are found in neonatal specimens as infants do not demonstrate anti-A and anti-B antibodies (IgM) at birth. They can have passively acquired maternal antibodies and these are usually IgG antibodies. Titers of anti-A and anti-B increase by 6 months of age.

  Resolution: Reverse grouping is not done in neonates.

- **Elderly:** Elderly patients demonstrate decreased reactivity in reverse grouping due to decrease in antibody production.
- *Pathologic causes:* **Congenital agammaglobulinemia, hypogammaglobulinemia and X-linked Wiskott-Aldrich syndrome** have low concentration of anti-A and anti-B antibodies.

  CLL, multiple myeloma, Waldenstrom's macroglobulinemia patients who are on immunosuppressive therapy or plasma exchange.

  Serum protein electrophoresis and immunoglobulin levels **should be done to** confirm the possibility of the diseases.
- **Bone marrow transplant:** Immunosuppression produces temporary hypogammaglobulinemia. These cases have reduced titers of ABO antibodies.
- **Prozoning:**
  1. Prozone phenomenon is associated with antibody excess. High antibody titers may not cause the agglutination of A or B cells, as all antigen sites are bound and visual agglutination is not produced.
  2. High titres of anti-A or anti-B are not detected due to steric hindrance by complement C1.

  Resolution: Repeat with a1:10 dilution of the serum with saline or 5 minutes incubation at room temperature.

Category III: Unexpected Antigen Reactions

- When strong serum group reactions are contradicted by weak antigen reactions of the same specificity, unexpected antigen reaction should be suspected.
- When an individual appears to be group AB, careful evaluation with auto controls, bovine albumin, etc. should be used for validation the result.

Causes of unexpected antigen reactions include:
- Polyagglutination
- Antibody coated red cells
- Acquired B antigens
- Rouleaux formation
- Multiple myeloma

- Waldenstrom's macroglobulinemia
- Plasma cell dyscrasiasis
- Wharton's jelly and serum separator tubes containing gels
- Chimerism
  Washing the cells, free of serum allows a valid cell typing.

	Antibodies			Cells			
	Anti-A	Anti-B	Anti-AB	A1	B	O	Auto
Unwashed RBCs	4+	2+	4+	2+	4+	2+	2+
Washed RBCs	4+	0	4+				
Saline replacement				0	4+	0	0

Note: In the above example, there is discrepancy with forward and reverse grouping and autocontol has reaction. With washed RBCs it is A blood group. Saline replacement disperses the rouleaux formation.

Antibody coated red cells can be found in following situations:
- Cold autoantibody
- Warm autoantibody
- Haemolytic transfusion reaction and HDN

Resolution: Washing red cells or warming tube to 37°C will disperse the agglutination.

Polyagglutination

Bacterial infection particularly due to Clostridium species exposes the hidden T antigen. This is due to the action of **bacterial neuraminidase** which removes sialic acid from the red cell surface.

These **Tn activated** cells are agglutinated by adult human anti-sera as they have antibody to this antigen, giving false positive results.

- Cells are agglutinated by ABO compatible adult human sera but not by cord sera.
- Due to IgM polyagglutinins present in normal adult sera.
- They react with abnormal membrane structure exposed by microbial enzymes (T, Tk, Th, VA) or a somatic mutation.

- Using monoclonal antisera can be used to obtain valid results.
- These antibodies can be classified using lectins.

	Antibodies			Cells			
	Anti-A	Anti-B	Anti-AB	A1	B	O	Auto
Polyclonal antisera	1+	1+	1+	4+	4+	0	0
Monoclonal antisera	0	0	0				

Note: Above example shows T-activation which fails to react with monoclonal sera.

Resolution:

1. Treat the cells with proteolytic enzymes before testing which can destroy Tn exposed RBCs.

2. Use monoclonal anti-sera to obtain valid results.

Acquired B Antigen

Patient with bacterial infections, often cancer of colon or rectum may have false B like antigen. Due to action of microbial enzymes causing deacetylation of A antigen or adsorption of bacterial polysaccharide. Removal of acetyl group, the N-acetyl galactosamine, resulting in galactosamine which crossreacts with anti-B giving the cells to appear as B cells (Fig. 18.1).

By altering the pH (lowering) of the anti-B reagent to the antigen–antibody reaction can be avoided.

Diagram to show acquired B antigen

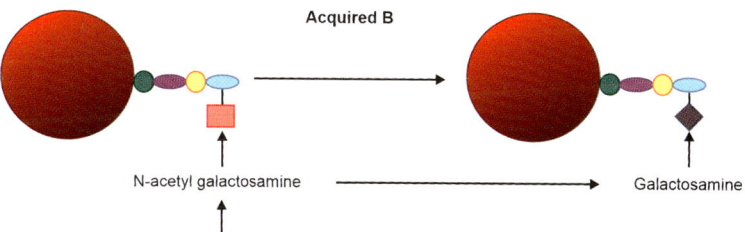

Bacteria having deacetylating enzyme splits A antigen resulting in acquired B antigen

Fig. 18.1: Formation of acquired B

Resolution:
1. Check the patient's diagnosis.
2. Test the patient's serum with his or her own red cells.
   No agglutination is seen if acquired B determinant is present, i.e. anti-B in the serum of acquired B person does not agglutinate autologous red cells.
3. Test the RBCs with monoclonal anti-B anti-sera.

The agglutination is fragile and easily dispersed

- *In vitro* immune complex attachment
  - Formed by dyes, drugs and reagents preservatives which get adsorbed onto the red cells. These are removed by washing the cells.
- Contaminating antibody in the sera
  - Anti-Yt, anti-Co antibodies to low incidence antigens
  - Repeat testing with a different lot of reagents gives valid results.

Agents causing non-specific agglutination

- **Serum separator tubes** containing gels may cause non-specific aggregation of red cells.
- **Wharton's jelly in cord blood:** Wharton's jelly in cord blood can trap the RBCs appearing like agglutination.

Resolution: Wash cells minimum two times before testing.
   Problems are less, if the blood sample is taken with needle and syringe.
   Using autologous controls, 6–8% albumin and washing the red cells with warm saline may yield a valid typing.

Chimerism

- This is temporary or genetic condition with simultaneous presence of two or more populations of red cells.
- Seen with
  - Intrauterine transfusion
  - Exchange transfusion
  - Allogenic bone marrow transplants
  - Feto-maternal haemorrhage
  - Dispermy
  - Mosiacism

Genetic chimerism: Exchange of hematopoietic tissue between fraternal twins.

Mosiacism: Occurs with dispermy when one ovum is fertilized by two sperms. Two populations of cells are recognised as self.

Category IV: Unexpected Antibody Reactions

- This is the most common cause of ABO discrepancies.
- Autologous controls and serum grouping with O cells are needed to detect the discrepancy.
- Causes include:
  - Rouleaux and pseudoagglutination
  - A subgroups with anti-A1 antibodies
  - Cold autoantibodies
  - Cold alloantibodies
  - Passively acquired anti-A or anti-B
- Rouleaux and pseudoagglutination: Elevated levels of globins from multiple myeloma, Waldenstrom's macroglobulinemia, elevated level of fibrinogen, high molecular weight expanders, etc.

  Resolution: True agglutination is stable in saline, whereas rouleaux and pseudoagglutination will disperse with saline
- A subgroup with anti-A1
  - Anti-A1 is found in 1–8% of A2 group individuals, 22–35% of A2B group individuals.
  - Anti-A1 antibodies are usually not reactive at 37°C, however, if reactive at 37°C, a compatible blood which is A1 negative should be issued.

	Antibodies			Cells					
	Anti-A	Anti-B	Anti-AB	Anti-A1	A1	A2	B	O	Auto
	4+	0	4+				4+	0	0
Additional test	4+	0	4+	0	2+	0	4+	0	0

Note: In this example, it is blood group A2 with anti-A1 antibodies, cold antibodies.

- Autoanti-I and anti-IH cause strong agglutination of all adult cells at room temperature.

- Warm saline washing of red cells gives valid results
- Cold alloantibodies
  - React with A1, B and O cells
  - An immediate spin reaction with group O screening cells is indicative of anti-M, anti-N, anti-P1
  - Autologous controls are negative
  - Repeat serum grouping with known M negative A1 and B cells.

| | Antibodies | | | Cells | | | | |
	Anti-A	Anti-B	Anti-AB	A1	B	O	Auto	Cord O
Unwashed RBCs	3+	4+	4+	4+	3+	3+	2+	1+
Washed RBCs	2+	4+	4+					
DTT	0+	4+	4+					
Auto-adsorbed serum				4+	0	0	0	0

Note: For IgM cold antibody (anti-I, H, M, N, P and Lewis), washing the cells with warm saline or dithiothreitol (DTT) or 2-mercaptoethenol treatment yields immunoglobulin free cells. **In the above example, it is B blood group with autoanti-I in serum.**

For IgG antibodies, using low protein reagents allow valid grouping. They can also be removed by 45°C elution or treatment with chloroquine diphosphate.

| Antibodies | | | | Cells | | | | |
Anti-A	Anti-B	Anti-AB	**Anti-H**	A1 cells	B cells	O cells	O cells (cord)	Auto
0	0	0	0	4+	4+	4+	4+	0

Note: No agglutination with anti-A, and anti-B antisera. It looks apparently as O blood group in forward blood grouping. In reverse grouping not only with A1, B cells, but also with O cells and O cord cells, agglutination is seen. There is no auto-agglutination. Anti-H lectin resolves the problem and this blood is of Bombay Blood group. If anti-H is added to any of the normal O, A, B or AB cells, they will agglutinate. Only Bombay blood group red cells will not show any agglutination.

Blood Bank Organization and its Management

Introduction

- Blood transfusion service (BTS) is a vital component of any health care delivery system.
- The aim of blood transfusion services should be to provide effective blood and blood products, which are safe as possible and adequate to meet patients' needs.
- A blood transfusion service is a complex organization, requiring careful designing and management.

National Blood Policy (2007)

A need for modification and changes in the blood transfusion service has necessitated formulation of National Blood Policy (2002, revision 2007).[32]

Objectives

1. To provide safe and adequate quantity of blood and blood components.
2. To make available adequate resources to develop and re-organize the BTS in the entire country.
3. To make latest technology available for operating the BTS and ensures its functioning in an updated manner.
4. To launch extensive awareness programmed for donor information, motivation, education, recruitment and retention in order to ensure adequate availability of safe blood.
5. To encourage appropriate clinical use of blood and blood products.

6. To strengthen the manpower through human resource development.
7. To encourage research and development in the field of transfusion medicine.
8. To take adequate regulatory and legislative steps for monitoring and evaluation of blood. Transfusion services and to take steps to eliminate profiteering in blood banks.

General Considerations for Setting Up a Blood Bank

- General guidelines
- Basic structure and designing of a blood bank
- Location
- Aims and operating policies
- Staffing pattern
- Personnel management

General Guidelines

- Location
  - Not exposed to strong sunshine
  - Proper natural lighting of rooms and protection from dust and insects
  - Adequate protection against rains and snow
  - Stand by generator
- Equipment and instruments for different sections
- Utilities—water, electricity, fuel
- Consumable supplies
- Lab reagents, bags, etc.
- Office supplies
- Quality control program followed in BTC
- Laboratory safety precautions
- Basic financial consideration and budgeting.

Building

- Located in hospital premises
- Provides easy access for donors and staff, allows quick and safe transportation of blood and components
- Well lighted, ventilated protected
- Away from sewage, drain or similar unhygienic surroundings.

Standard Floor Space Requirement

Standard floor space shall cover a minimum area of 100 sq.m. for whole blood collection and an additional area of 50 sq.m. for component preparation.

Donor Area

- Reception and donor waiting area
  - Spacious
  - Well ventilated
  - Proper and comfortable sitting arrangement
  - Social worker or technical staff to answer queries and alleviate anxiety
- Medical examination room
- Donor refreshment-cum-resting room
- Should have AC with proper and comfortable seating
- Drinking water and refreshments
- Observation room

Medical Examination Room

- Jar with copper sulphate
- Sterile lancet and swabs, spirit
- Capillary tubes with rubber bulb

Blood Donation/Collection Room

- Should have AC, proper light, washable floors
- Should not be visible for people in waiting room
- Should have comfortable beds
- Sterile equipment
- Refrigerators and resuscitation equipment
- Dust free, quite and pleasant with privacy for recording history and examination
- Should have emergency drugs
- Connected to reception on one side and refreshment room on other

Equipment in Blood Donation Room

- Donor beds, chairs and tables
- Bedside table

- Sphygmomanometer and stethoscope
- Clinical thermometer
- Disposable blood collection bags and sets: 3 types
  - 350 mL with 49 mL CPD-A1 anticoagulant (single bag)
  - 450 mL with 63 mL CPD-A1 anticoagulant (double bag)
  - 450 mL with 63 mL CPD-A1 anticoagulant (triple bag).
- PVC sterile bags, easy to store with attached tubing and needle.
- Disposable needles and syringes.
- Shaking apparatus for proper mixing of blood and anti-coagulant.
- Blood bag weighing scale.
- Heat sealer or tube sealer artery forceps and scissors.
- Test tubes for typing and serological testing.
- Emergency drugs: Adrenaline, corticosteroids, metachlopro-mide, dextrose, normal saline, etc.
- Oxygen cylinders with mask gauges and pressure regulators.
- Cotton, sterile gauge, antiseptic solution and adhesive tapes.

Laboratory

Should be spacious, AC with proper lighting.

Samples are processed for grouping and crossmatching; blood is issued accordingly.

Equipment Used in Laboratory

- Microscope, centrifuge, water baths
- Refrigerators
- Incubators
- Graduated pipettes, glass slides, test tubes
- Test tube racks of different specifications
- Wash bottles, plain and EDTA vials

Refrigerator

- Tested and untested blood stored separately with constant temperature of 2–6°C.
- Digital dial thermometer, recording thermograph and alarm device.
- Constant power supply.

Cleaning, Sterilization and Other Rooms

- Divided into 2 portions:
  1. Washing area
  2. Sterilization area (with autoclave and distillation plant)
- Administrative room, doctor's room and cleaner's room
- Office: Telephone, card index cabinets, filing cabinets, computer with printer, stationary, donor registration card
- Accessories
- Reagents:
  - Standard blood group sera-anti-A, anti-B, anti-AB with known controls
  - Rh typing sera
  - Anti-human globulin (Coombs' test)
  - Bovine albumin
  - ELISA test kits for hepatitis, HIV and malaria, syphilis

Infrastructure

- Water: Adequate, round the clock, uncontaminated
- Electricity: Reliable supply and powerful standby generator
- Sewage
- Communication system

Staff

Medical officers: 2

With MD degree in pathology with suitable experience in transfusion med (or as per the guidelines of drugs controller, India).

Technicians: 11

A degree/diploma in medical laboratory technology with at least 6 months of training. They can also perform a role of phlebotomist.

Registered nurse: 1

Attend donor and perform phlebotomy

Technical supervisor: 1

- In blood bank where components are prepared

- Degree/diploma medical laboratory technology with 1 yr experience in preparation and handling of blood and blood components

Public relation/information personnel: 1

To answer queries, motivate donors, educate them and alleviate their anxiety

Lab assistants:	2
Cleaner:	1
Secretary/clerk-cum-typist:	1
Record keeper:	1

Note: Staffing for blood bank varies according to workload and this is the minimum staffing for 1000–5000 blood units collection per year.

Waste Disposal

Bag colour	Type of waste
Yellow	Human anatomical waste, lab cultures
Red	Material contaminated with blood, non-sharp disposable items, gloves, catheters, tubes, IV sets
Blue or white	Needles, syringes, scalpels, blades, broken glasses
Black	Discarded medicines

Non-infectious Material is Recycled

Biodegradable waste

- Landfill
- Vermiculture
- Buried

Infectious solid waste

- Incinerated

Infectious liquid waste

- Disinfected
- Flushed out

Component Separation Room

- Units of whole blood are separated into various components and stored at optimal conditions.
- Area has to be 50 sq m.
- Completely secluded, sterile with restricted entry.
- With AC, temperature of 20–25°C.
- Well equipped with refrigerators, deep freezers, etc.

Advantages of blood components

- Enable selective transfusion of blood products according to specific needs.
- Allow optimal survival of each of the components.
- Maximizes the number of transfusion recipients.
- Enables blood collection agencies to maximize their financial returns.

Following are the components

- Packed red cells
- Fresh frozen plasma
- Platelet rich plasma
- Platelet concentrates
- Cryoprecipitate
- Cryo-poor plasma
- Granulocyte concentrate

Equipment in component separation room

- Plasma expressor
- Refrigerated centrifuge
- Dielectric sealer
- Weighing device
- Refrigerator
- Platelet agitator with incubator (+20°C)
- Deep freezer (–30°C to –60°C)
- Cell separator

Refrigerator

- To keep processed blood like packed red cells and whole blood
- Should have capacity to store 210 bags of 450 mL capacity

- Maintain constant temperature
- 4–6°C+/– 2°C
- Attached digital dial thermometer
- Continuous power supply

Deep freezer
- Maintaining temperature of –30° to –60°C
- 500 liters capacity
- Store fresh frozen plasma and cryoprecipitate

Platelet rotator/agitator
- Provide constant gentle agitation
- Room temperature
- Store platelet concentrates

Standard Operating Procedures (SOPs)

Maintenance of written standard operating procedures (SOPs) which include all steps to be followed in collection, processing, compatibility testing, storage of blood and/or preparation of components.
- Written by blood bank director
- Reviewed and revised every year
- These minimize the human mistakes

Note: Also refer to Quality Improvement and Quality Control in Blood Transfusion.

Medicolegal Concerns and Ethical Aspects

Blood transfusion services in a blood bank have high potential risk of adverse reactions to recipients and high risk of legal liability to hospital.

Risks include
- Acceptance of donor
- Extraction of blood
- Storage of blood and its derivative
- Procedures like grouping, crossmatching
- Transfusion to the donor

Documentation and Record Maintenance

- To judge the performance of blood bank
- To trace any unit of blood from its source to final position
- In legal or investigation process
- Compilation of statistical data of performance monthly and yearly
- Written as well as computerized documentation and records should be maintained.

Various records to be maintained

- Blood donor record including rare donor panels, donor referrals and donor reactions
- Master records
- Issue register
- Records of blood bags
- Transfusion adverse reaction records
- Recipient's register
- Blood stock register
- Register of blood grouping and crossmatching
- Register for grouping and typing of OPD and ward patients
- Records of apparatus, reagents, etc.
- Quality control records
- Patient/recipient's record
- Attendance registers for staff

Quality Assurance

- Customer focused, strategic and systemic approach to continuous improvement involving all persons in the organization.
- Provides opportunity for all staff to be a part of team approach.
- Provides common structure for improvement of problems and processes.
- Customer needs to be satisfied with quality services, on time and at best possible cost.

Quality Control

- Testing routinely performed to ensure proper functioning of materials, equipment and methods.

- QC performance characteristics and acceptable ranges should be readily available for the prompt detection and appropriate handling of unacceptable variations.
- A separate QC department and medical officer should take appropriate actions.
- It includes:
  - Proper construction of premises
  - Continuous monitoring of the equipment
  - Competence of the personnel
  - Testing of defined number of units of each product for appropriate parameters
  - When unfavorable results—procedures must be reviewed and appropriate measures taken
  - Proper documentation and record maintenance

According to Drugs and Cosmetics Act it is mandatory that in any storage equipment in the blood bank the following are a must:
- Digital display of temperature inside
- Thermograph
- Alarm system
- Temperature of the thermometer should be compared periodically to the temperature on the recording chart
- A difference of more than 2°C is not acceptable.

Accreditation

Laboratory accreditation is a procedure by which an authoritative body gives formal recognition that a laboratory is competent to carry out specific tasks based on third party assessment. Emphasis is on technical competence which also includes quality system management
- Currently **Drugs and Cosmetic Rules under Government of India,**[33] provide accreditation services for blood bank.
- With the national blood policy now in place, the government is all set to take the next step towards improving transfusion services in the country.
- National Aids Control Organization (NACO)[34] plans to come up with an accreditation programmed for blood banks, blood storage centers and other centers involved in providing transfusion services.

Worldwide accreditations for blood banks

- Food and Drug Administration (FDA)
- American Association of Blood Banks (AABB)
- College of American Pathologists (CAP)
- National Committee for Clinical Laboratory Standards (NCCLS)

Legislation

- India has a procedure for mandatory licensing under the *Drugs and Cosmetics Rules* for blood banks.
- Any blood bank can function only if it qualifies the criteria laid down by the organization.
- These range from quality and variety of the equipment used, to the qualification of the working staff, source of procurement of blood and blood components to labeling of blood units/components licensing is renewed every year if transfusion center fulfils all specifications.

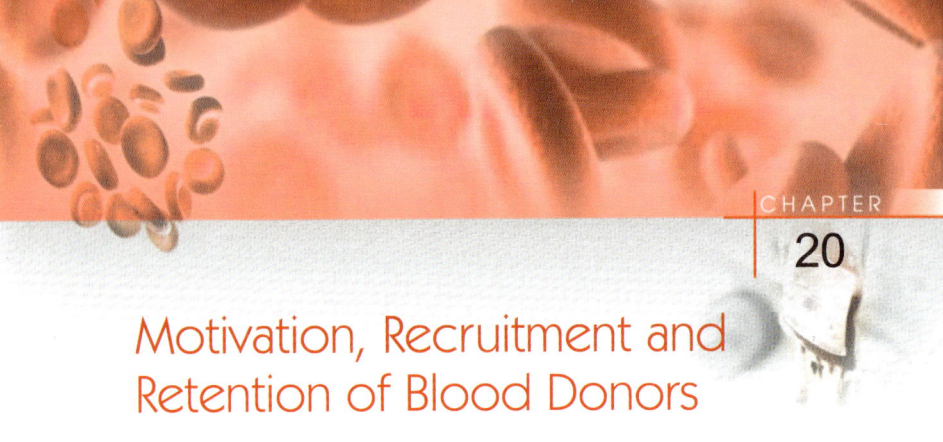

Motivation, Recruitment and Retention of Blood Donors

Blood cannot be manufactured. For continuous supply of blood and its products, blood has to come from generous donations from blood donors. To ensure a safe and adequate supply of blood and blood products motivation, recruitment, selection and retention of voluntary non-remunerated blood donors are of at most importance. The first step towards blood safety is to encourage blood donations from **voluntary** and **non-remunerated low-risk** blood donors. Blood from a voluntary, repeat and regular donor is the best. **A regular donor is one who donates blood two to three times a year and continues to donate at least once a year.** Voluntary non-remunerated regular blood donors who donate blood out of self sacrifice are considered safe blood donors. In many countries, **continuous efforts are needed to achieve 100% voluntary blood donation**. It is well established that paid donors constitute a group with high-risk behaviour leading to greater chances of transfusion-transmitted infections in the recipients. If the blood replacement system is in use, it is necessary to impose strict vigilance to identify paid donors.

Donor Motivation

While planning **donor education and motivation campaign**, the following should be kept in mind:
- People do not donate blood unless they are asked to donate.
- There are sufficient potential donors available.
- There are several myths and misconceptions about blood donation in the public.

Education therefore is an important bridge between awareness and recruitment. Donor education is essential to ensure recruitment of safe donors.

Essential Steps in Donor Motivation

This is done by the following ways:

- Appeal for blood donation through lectures and focused group discussion.
- Continued motivation and education of potential donors.
- Involving important public figures and community leaders in blood donation education programmes.
- Retention of safe donors.
- Organizing donor recruitment campaigns on a continuous basis.
- **Developing messages:** A clear and simple message conveyed in a local language is most effective. **All health education or communication materials,** e.g. posters, leaflets, flip charts, etc., once prepared, **should be field-tested** among a subset of target population and suitably modified based on the feedback from the field test. Educational material suitable for the target group should then be prepared and used for the purpose of motivating potential donors. Traditional media, such as songs, folk dance, street plays, puppetry, etc. can prove valuable, especially in rural settings. The local community groups and youth groups can participate actively in preparation as well as in the use of such promotional material.
- **Communication approaches:** Methods and approaches to be employed for communication or awareness programme could include the use of mass media—newspapers, radio and television; interpersonal communication through person-to-person interaction; group educational workshops, e.g. lectures, exhibition—posters and banners; use of celebrities to convey messages; regular contact with potential donors through greeting cards, phone calls, blood donation drives on important national days, recognition of regular blood donors, etc.

Proper and effective communication strategy can help to motivate potential donors to become donors, encourage suitable donors to be regular donors, and discourage unsuitable individuals from donating blood, thus reducing the chances of transmitting infections through blood transfusion.

The main messages which the communication programme should highlight include the following:

- Target populations to be addressed may include:
  - Youth above the age of 18 years in colleges
  - People at workplaces, i.e. factory workers, office workers, etc.
  - General population
  - Organizers of blood donation campaigns
  - Religious and community leaders
- Need for preventing transfusion-transmitted infections and risk associated with blood collected from paid blood donors.
- Assuring harmlessness of blood donation, safety of blood donors through their pre-donation medical checkup and use of disposable equipment for blood collection.
- Community responsibility for blood donation.
- Information about collection, processing and supply of blood.
- Blood as a life savior to the needy and emergency cases.
- Blood donation through organized group or individual recruitment.
- Organizing and providing infrastructure.

Donor education and information materials, donor questionnaires and consent forms should be prepared in simple language and translated for use according to regional variations. Picture presentations or flip charts can be used to educate donors who cannot read printed educational material.

For satisfactory donor recruitment, the first essential step is to initiate knowledge, attitude and practice studies among a sample of donors and non-donors. The objective is to understand donor demographic profiles as well as the prevailing misconceptions, beliefs and fears leading to a negative attitude towards blood donation. This should also cover socio-economic and cultural factors relating to blood donations, such as asking donors how they decided to donate or learnt about the donation centers. The information so obtained could be helpful in developing appropriate messages to be used during recruitment of campaigns, creating and strengthening positive attitudes towards blood donation, and developing and implementing focused awareness programmes for target populations.

Planning of education and motivation campaigns should take into consideration the profile of the target audience in terms of socio-economic and cultural background, age group, sex, level of education as well as physical, environmental and other factors.

Retaining Donors

To increase the number of voluntary blood donors and retain them as regular donors, efforts are being made by most of the blood banks. This is important because **the prevalence of infections in regular donors is known to be much lower than in new donors**. Recruiting regular blood donors will help in increasing the yield of plasma for therapeutic and fractionation purposes. The regular donors are tested each time they donate, which further increases the safety of blood. For an effective donor retention programme, building a long-term relationship with donors is crucial. **Following are some of the measures that may help in donor retention:**

- To have a clean and easily accessible location for blood donation.
- Time schedule convenient to most of the donors.
- Donors should be given personal attention.
- They should not be made to wait long.
- Staff behaviour is perhaps the most important factor. The staff should therefore be courteous, trained and experienced in providing proper donor care.
- The staff should make the procedure of blood donation a pleasant and comfortable experience.

- The donors must be appreciated and thanked for their contribution and assured of total confidentiality.
- Appropriate follow-up and medical support would go a long way in donor retention.

According to blood transfusion safety department of essential health technologies of World Health Organization, high priority should be given to the **elimination** of family/replacement and paid blood donor systems, which are associated with a significantly higher prevalence of TTIs. Voluntary non-remunerated blood donors from low-risk populations who give blood regularly are the foundation of a safe and adequate blood supply. **Important activities include**:

- Appointment of an officer responsible for the **national blood donor programme.**
- Establishment of a BTS unit responsible for donor education, motivation, recruitment and retention.
- Appointment of a **designated blood donor recruitment officer.**
- Preparation of SOPs in accordance with BTS guidelines.
- Training of staff in the blood donor unit.
- Identification of **donor populations at risk for TTIs.**
- Development of **educational materials.**
- Establishment of a **register of voluntary non-remunerated blood donors.**
- Assurance of safe blood collection procedures, including donor selection and deferral, donor care and confidentiality.

Ensuring Safety during Blood Donations

During blood donation campaigns, it is crucial to ensure the safety of the donors. The donor should willingly consent to donate blood without being pressurised. The organizers of donation campaigns should be discouraged from offering expensive incentives to blood donors. Information and counselling are essential for enhancing donor awareness, perception, motivation, self-deferral and recall. The donor should be assured of absolute confidentiality. Moreover, the procedure for blood collection should be made completely safe, e.g. by using disposable needles, syringes and blood collection packs to instill confidence in the donors about their own safety.

Donor Record Maintenance

A well-maintained donor record, kept in strict confidentiality, is an essential part of the programme. It is helpful in donor retention as well as in tracing the donor for any specific needs, such as requirement of rare blood group, donor recall in case of post-transfusion infection, confirmation of test results and counseling.

Recent Advances in Blood Banking

Virtual Blood Bank[35,36]

Virtual blood bank (online blood bank) is the computer-controlled, electronically linked information management system that allows **online ordering and real-time**, remote delivery of blood for transfusion. It connects the **site of testing to the point of care** at a remote site in a real-time fashion with networked computers thus maintaining the integrity of immuno-hematology test results. It has taken the advantages of information and communication technologies to ensure the accuracy of patient, specimen and blood component identification and to enhance personnel traceability and system security. The built-in logics and process constraints in the design of the virtual blood bank can guide the selection of appropriate blood and minimize transfusion risk. The quality of blood inventory is ascertained and monitored, and an audit trail for critical procedures in the transfusion process is provided by the **paperless system**.

Thus, the **virtual blood bank** can help to ensure that the right patient receives the right amount of the right blood component at the right time.

Computer crossmatch is considered safer or more efficient system than the antiglobulin and immediate spin crossmatch, provided that the ABO and Rh typing has been done twice and patient has no history of clinically significant antibodies.

Barcode Scanning

Barcode scanning can serve as an adjunct to manual checking and is prompt to take the operator through each step of patient identification. Major problems related to the use of barcoded identification bracelet are: (A) the availability of equipment (barcode scanner and printer) at each point of care, (B) the need to remove the identification bracelet for patient treatment, such as during surgery.

It is important to note that electronic control of the transfusion process can only help to reduce, but not totally eliminate, human errors. It should never replace human thinking and should be treated only as an adjunct to manual checking and verification. For non-emergency transfusion, group-identical and electronically crossmatched donor units will be issued for patients with a negative antibody screen.

The system will prevent the allocation of ABO non-identical blood and check the concordance of ABO typing results tested on different specimens and/or at different occasions.

For patients with specific transfusion requirements such as those with irregular antibodies, only designated donor units will be issued (the designated donor units may have been delivered and stored in a remote refrigerator or they will have to be collected from the central blood bank).

The expiry date of the donor unit is checked before its release, and some systems can allocate donor unit closest to the end of its shelf life.

Radio frequency identification device (RFID):[37,38] RFID technology systems utilize radio frequency electromagnetic fields to obtain data for tracking and identifying medical products and goods. The two main components of RFID are tags and readers. The tags consist of silicon microchips and antennas that receive or emit radiofrequency waves.

RFIDs contain identification tags that enable scanning a device (reader) so contents, location, manufactured date, order numbers, batch numbers, dosage information and shipping data can be transmitted to a corresponding data terminal. In healthcare organizations, tags have been placed on patients, pharmaceuticals, mobile assets, and blood products. RFID technology offers several benefits with regard to blood bank product management, including decreased transfusion errors, reduction of product loss, and more efficient inventory management. Barriers to RFID implementation include the cost associated with system implementation and patient privacy issues. Implementation of an RFID system can be a significant investment. However, when observing the positive impact that such systems may have on transfusion safety and inventory management, the cost associated with RFID systems can easily be justified.

RFID in blood bank inventory management is vital to ensure efficient product inventory management and positive patient outcomes.

Immunocamouflage Technique to Develop Universal RBCs

Scientists have discovered a way to avoid issuing wrong blood type and can serve as all-purpose red blood cells. To develop universal red blood cells, the red cells are covered with a multi-layered polymer shell of polyethylene glycol such that the antigenic sites are not identified by the body's immune mechanism.

Smart Blood Bag Management System[38]

Blood has to be kept at fixed temperature during transportation. 3T (time, temperature and tracking) enhanced system to provide necessary temperature and to prevent mismatch of blood a smart blood bag box using sensor network in the blood bank and RFID sensor tag is placed on the blood bag. This system can sense the change and also record the time. Also patient information will be available with unique ID, correct identification of blood bag, thus, error can be prevented in transfusion of required specific blood.

Unused Donor Units

Unused donor units can be returned to the remote refrigerator through the BBLIS. The time when the donor unit leaves the refrigerator will be recorded, and it will be barred from re-issue if the donor unit is returned after 30 min. This will safeguard the integrity of the donor unit and prevent bacterial overgrowth and other problems associated with inappropriate storage.

The Blood Vending Machine

A latest addition to the virtual blood bank is the blood vending machine. The machine consists of two components: (A) An intelligent temperature-controlled blood storage and dispensing refrigerator with computerized controlled electromagnetic door lock and (B) An attached kiosk that is a purpose-built computer terminal with identity card reader and barcode scanner for personnel login and patient identification, process control and compatibility label printing.

The refrigerator contains a rotating carousel with individually electronically controlled and lockable compartments for undesignated donor units of each ABO group and one compartment for reserved and serologically crossmatched donor units, which enable physical and electronic control of access, allocation and dispensing of group-identical electronically crossmatched or reserved serologically crossmatch-compatible donor units.

The blood vending machine allows bidirectional informatics connectivity and ensures that: (A) Only authorized personnel can gain access, (B) Expiry date of donor unit is checked, (C) Validity of reserved unit is confirmed, (D) Oldest available donor unit is dispensed and (E) Inventory and temperature are monitored continuously by the central blood bank.

The donor unit will be automatically assigned and dispensed by the refrigerator and labeled at the kiosk. It has further enhanced the safety, efficacy and security of the virtual blood bank as it limits access to only the correct donor units, reduces donor unit expiry and provides an audit trail for the personnel involved and procedures undertaken. The stock can be replenished at the convenience of the blood bank staff who will be alerted when the inventory falls below a pre-set limit. An obstacle to the wider use of such a blood vending machine is probably its cost, which is, at present, several times that of the usual blood storage refrigerator.

Blood transfusion is a high-risk process because of the complexity of its many procedures (from blood sampling to laboratory testing and blood administration) and the involvement of multiple staff from different departments.

The virtual blood bank has taken the full advantage of computer crossmatch, i.e. immediate availability of compatible blood without the need of prior allocation of donor units to designated patients, and has allowed the controlled use of group-identical blood, real-time inventory monitoring and early stock replenishment.

The use of barcode or other identification devices can eliminate human errors in data transcription. Electronic process control can help ensure compliance with transfusion guidelines and regulatory requirements.

The advent of information technology has enabled us to come closer to the goal of zero-risk, zero-time-lag and zero-wastage transfusion—a goal that was only a dream in the past but might be reachable in the not-so-distant future.

Recent Advances in Platelet Transfusion

The demand for platelet transfusions continues to grow. Several complementary approaches may help to meet this demand in the future. First, platelet bacterial testing is beginning to allow the extension of platelet storage beyond 5 days.

Studies are also underway aimed at better preserving viability and function during *ex vivo* platelet storage: Additive solutions and other approaches are being developed.

Bacterial Testing[34-36]

The BacT/ALERT automated blood culture system, can be used to screen platelet concentrates for bacterial growth.

Platelet products production of CO_2 are generally sampled on day 1 after collection. The samples are cultured for a period of time, typically 24 hours, and if the cultures fail to produce abnormal levels of CO_2, the product is released into inventory.

Both aerobic and anaerobic cultures may be performed, although it is known that aerobic organisms cause the vast majority of septic reactions.

Current generation rapid bacterial tests have a turn around time of a few hours or less, and use <1 mL of platelet product. They have a lower sensitivity than culture, however, on the order of 10^3–10^4 CFU/mL.

In principle, rapid bacterial tests could be used for quality control, as an adjunct to another test, e.g. initial culture, or as a standalone release test.

Licensing criteria for rapid bacterial tests are being developed by the FDA.

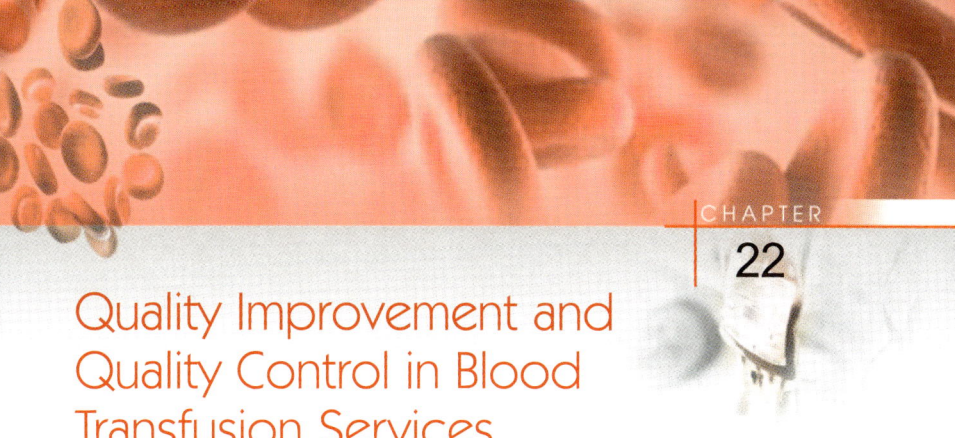

Quality Improvement and Quality Control in Blood Transfusion Services

Blood transfusion service is a vital part of the national health service and there is no substitute for human blood and its components. Increasing advancement in the field of transfusion technology has necessitated enforcing strict control over the quality of blood and its products.

Definition of Quality

"Quality is degree of excellence" or superiority of kind. According to WHO definition, quality is "the consistent and reliable performance of services or products in conformity with specified standards". In the patient's view, the quality of service is "free of defects and results free of faults".

Quality Assurance (QA)

The term QA is for all measures from recruitment of donor to transfusion of blood and blood products. This includes pre-analytical, analytical and post-analytical processes. The objective of QA is to achieve precision and accuracy. With QA the efficiency and effectiveness of blood bank is enhanced.

Quality Control (QC)

QC is integral part of QA. QC is:
1. Management of testing process
2. Assessment of accuracy and reproducibility of the test
3. Equipment and instrument monitoring
4. Reagent testing
5. Quality of blood and blood products

The blood bank professionals come across quality of standards set by variety of agencies that tend to have different objectives.

The Joint Commission for Accreditation of Healthcare Organization (JCAHO) focuses on service aspects, examination of components of transfusion services involved in ordering, processing and transfusion of blood.

The US Food and Drug Administration (FDA) in America, recommends testing for 7 infectious diseases including *Trypanosoma cruzi* and West Nile virus.

In order to improve the standards of blood and its components, the central government through Drugs Controller General of India has formulated a comprehensive legislation to ensure better quality control system on collection, storage, testing and distribution of blood and its components. Central government amended from time to time the existing requirements of blood banks in the Drugs and Cosmetics Act, 1940 and rules thereunder to meet the latest standards.

National Blood Policy[32]

Government of India published the national blood policy in the year 2002, later again revised in 2007. The objectives of the policy is to provide safe, adequate quantity of blood, blood components and products. The main aim of the policy is to procure non-remunerated regular blood donors by the blood banks. The policy also addresses various issues with regard to technical personnel, research, development and to eliminate profiteering by the blood banks by selling blood. The policy also envisages that fresh licences to stand alone blood banks in private sector shall not be granted and renewal of such blood banks shall be subjected to thorough scrutiny.

Note: Refer to topic on "blood bank organization and its management".

National Accreditation Board for Hospitals and Healthcare (NABH)

NABH offers accreditation services to hospitals and blood banks. Accreditation of blood banks/blood centers and blood transfusion services by NABH strives to improve quality and safety of collecting, processing, testing, transfusion and distribution of blood and blood products. It assesses the quality and operational systems in place within the facility.

National AIDS Control Organization (NACO)[34]

In order to improve the standards of blood banks and the blood transfusion services in our country, National AIDS Control Organization through Technical Resource Group on Blood Safety, **NACO,** Ministry of Health and Family Welfare Government of India, New Delhi **in 2007** has formulated comprehensive standards to ensure better quality control system on collection, storage, testing and distribution of blood and its components.

The objectives of NACO are the following:

- To bring about zero transmission of AIDS
- Blood safety program encouraged
- Only licensed blood banks allowed to operate in India
- Voluntary blood donation encouraged
- **Zonal blood testing centers** to be established which test the samples of blood for blood banks and report HIV results on the same day.

Blood as a Drug

The problems of transfusion associated acquired immunodeficiency syndrome resulted in a notification in 1989 under the Drugs and Cosmetics Act which made the test for HIV mandatory. The Drugs and Cosmetics Rules were again amended (Rules 68A, Part XB and Part XIIB of Schedule F) in the year 1992-93 and the DCGI was vested with the power of central licence approving authority (CLAA) to approve the license of notified drugs, viz blood and blood products, IV fluids, vaccines and sera.

Human blood is covered under the definition of "Drugs" under Section 2(b) of Drugs and Cosmetics Act. Hence, it is imperative that the blood banks need to be regulated under the Drugs and Cosmetics Act and Rules thereunder and the licence is granted for operating a blood bank by the State and Central Licensing Approving Authorities after inspection. Since blood and blood products are drugs, license is required for blood transfusion under Section 18 (c) of the said Act.

Continuous Quality Improvement (CQI)

This is based on view, that despite the almost care, processes and systems may not be perfectly correct. Procedures to identify these deviations have to be incorporated, such as:

1. Validation
2. QC
3. QA audit
4. Errors
5. Accidents
6. Complaints
7. Transfusion reactions.

These deviations are to be documented, investigated to find the root cause and corrective actions have to be taken.

The main components of quality in blood transfusion services involve the following components:

1. Organizational management
2. Infrastructure space instruments
3. Reagents and materials
4. Resources: Personnel, training and development
5. SOPs
6. Donors
7. Phlebotomy
8. Blood and blood products quality requirements
9. Safety in laboratory
10. Quality assurance
11. Internal and external quality control
12. Internal audit
13. Documentation

Organizational Management

For effective quality system, commitment and support from management is required at all levels including financial assistance.

Space and Instruments or Equipment

Space and instruments or equipment should be as per requirement by the guidelines.

For space, for blood and components please refer to chapter on "blood bank organization and its management".

Equipment

The equipment should have the record of the following:
1. Installation and verification documents
2. Calibration and maintenance schedule
3. Daily QC
4. Temperature and humidity monitoring
5. Breakdown follow-up

Calibration is a procedure done to know the performance and efficiency of the equipment by comparing/testing against a standardized equipment, so as to ensure the quality and safety of the product produced/stored.

Each instrument should have record of:
1. Frequency for performance checking
2. Record of every major repair
3. Traceability records

The standard equipment used for calibration should have traceability certificate by National Institute of Standards and Technology (NIST), issued from time to time.

The instrument should also undergo:

1. Safety checks

Safety of electrical equipment includes the intrinsic safety of the equipment and safety of its operations.

Majority of problems involving medical equipment are caused by improper use of the equipment and failure to install it correctly or not maintaining it satisfactorily.

All essential equipment in blood banks should have full backup of emergency electric supply.

2. Corrective measures

If any equipment is not functioning properly, the results of tests/products produced/stored are affected. So, corrective

TABLE 22.1: Calibration frequency for instruments in blood banks

Equipment	Performance	Frequency for performance checking	Minimum frequency of calibration
Temperature recorder (display)	Compare against calibrated thermometer	Daily	Once in 6 months
Deep storage		Daily	
Refrigerated centrifuge	Observe speed, temperature and time	Each day of use	Once a year
Haematocrit centrifuge	Observe speed, temperature and time	—	
General lab centrifuge	Observe speed, temperature and time		
Haemoglobino-meter standard	Standardized against cyanmethemoglobin	Each day of use	Once a year
Blood bank refrigerator	Standardized against known calibrated weight	Each day of use	
Blood bag weighing machine	Container of known calibrated weight	Each day of use	
Refractometer		Each day of use	
Water bath	Observe temperature	Each day of use	
Autoclave	Observe temperature and pressure	Each day of use	
Serological rotators	Control for correct results	Each day of use	
Laboratory thermometer	—		Before initial use and every 6 months
Digital thermometer	—		Before initial use and every 6 months
Blood agitator	Observe weight of first blood filled container for correct results	Every 15 days	Once a year
Platelet agitator		Each day of use	Once in 6 months
Automated blood cell counter	Known controls	Daily	
Pipettes	Volume	Once in a month	Once a year
Incubator	Temperature		Once a year
Stop watch	Time		

measures are to be taken without fail. The person in charge should identify the problem and suitable corrective steps have to be taken. The manufacturer may be contacted for regular and speedy repair.

Blood bank refrigerator
- Should be kept in clean and well-lit place.
- Should have continuous and stable power supply.
- Do not keep anything other than blood in the refrigerator.
- Record the temperature daily.
- Should have alarm system with periodic checkup.
- Calibration should be once in 12 months.

Standard thermometer
- Is used to compare laboratory thermometer daily.
- Should be calibrated once a year.
- Should have traceability certificate.
- Calibrated thermometers are necessary for checking the temperature to assess the functioning of refrigerators, water baths, incubators, etc.

BP apparatus: To be calibrated.

Reagents and materials
- Before choosing suppliers for reagents, evaluate the authenticity.
- Acceptance and rejection criteria of reagents should be viewed.
- Inventory should be maintained.
- Lot to lot verification should be done.
- Daily quality control should be run.
- They should be of good quality with minimum shelf life of one year.
- Reagents should be checked daily for their specificity and avidity, using known positive and negative controls.
- Reagents to be checked for appearance, turbidity and discoloration. Those reagents suggesting contamination should be discarded. Manufacturer's insert should specify titer, avidity and all other relevant information.

- At any given time, there should be two different batches of each reagent available—either from two different manufacturers or two different batches from the same manufacturer. These should be used for positive samples.
- All reagents should be checked for expiry date, and properly/clearly labeled. Instructions for use should be in the form of SOPs.
- Use positive and negative controls.
- Reagents should be kept at 4–6°C and never be frozen or follow manufacturer's instructions.
- Storage, supply and transportation of kits and reagents should be as per manufacturer's instructions.

TABLE 22.2: Frequency of testing reagents and solutions in blood bank	
Reagents and solutions	*Frequency of testing with controls*
Anti-human globulin sera	
Blood grouping sera	Each day of use
Lectins	
Red cells for serum grouping	
Reagents used for TTDs (Hepatitis B, C, HIV1 and 2, syphilis, malaria)	Each run
Normal saline (LISS and PBS)	Each day of use
Bovine albumin	

Quality Control of Reagents

Anti-human globulin (AHG) reagent

- One vial from every new batch should be checked for its specificity and reactivity using (incomplete anti-Rh) IgG coated cells.
- Each test should include positive and negative controls.
- Non-sensitized A, B and O cells should be checked to rule out non-specific reactions.
- All negative AHG tests should be confirmed by addition of IgG coated cells in the test. IgG coated cells should give positive agglutination.

Quality control of bovine albumin

- The reagent should be free of the non-specific agglutination and should not react with saline suspension of A, B and O cells.
- Reagent should give positive reaction with Rh(D) positive cells coated with incomplete anti-Rh(D) antibodies.

Quality control of red cells (control red cells) used for testing

- Cells should be prepared daily and should be free of haemolysis. There should be a pool of 3 individual cells for each group.
- Each batch of reagent cells (A, B and O) for serum grouping prepared should be tested to confirm specificity.

Red cell panel

- These are either commercially available or prepared in house. The red cells should be stored frozen, or at 4°C.
- Red cells stored for more than 48 hours at 4°C, should be checked for reactivity.

TABLE 22.3: Quality control of red cells		
Parameter	*Quality requirement*	*Frequency*
Appearance	No haemolysis or turbidity in supernatant by visual inspection	Daily
Reactivity and specificity	Positive reaction with known sera against red blood cell antigens	

Quality control of ABO anti-seras and anti-D anti-seras

- **Avidity:** Denotes the speed of reaction for visual agglutination and overall binding strength of anti-sera (antibodies).
- **Specificity:** Denotes clear-cut reaction with RBCs bearing the corresponding and no reaction with negative controls.
- **Potency (Titer):** It denotes strength of the reagent. It is the highest dilution of the anti-sera of which the macroscopic agglutination is seen.
- **Titration method:** Doubling dilution (1:2, 1:4, 1:8, 1:16, 1:32, 1:64, 1:128, 1:256, 1:512, 1:1024).

TABLE 22.4: Quality control of ABO reagents (anti-A, anti-B and anti-AB reagents)

Parameter	Quality requirement	Frequency
Appearance	No turbidity, precipitate, particles or gel formation by visual inspection	Daily and with new lot/batch
Specificity	Positive reaction with known sera against red blood cell antigens and no reaction with negative controls	
Avidity	Macroscopic agglutination with 50% red cell suspension in homologous serum/normal saline using slide test; 10 secs anti-A, anti-B and anti-AB with A1 and B cells at room temperature, 20 secs with A2 and A2B cells	
Reactivity	No immune haemolysis, rouleaux formation or prozone	
Potency	Undiluted serum should give +++ reactions in saline with 3% red cells suspension at room temperature, titre of 1:256 for anti-A, anti-B and anti-AB with A1 and B cells and 1:64 for A2 and A2B cells	Daily and with new lot/batch

TABLE 22.5: Acceptable titers and avidity and intensity of ABO blood group reagents

Anti-sera	Type of reagent	Type of cells	Titer	Avidity	Intensity
Anti-A	Polyclonal	A1	1:256	10–12 secs	+++
		A2	1:128	15–16 secs	++/+++
		A2B	1:64	15–18secs	++
	Monoclonal	A1	1:256	3–4 secs	+++
		A2	1:128	5–6 secs	++/+++
		A2B	1:64	5–6 secs	++++
Anti-B	Polyclonal	B	1:256	10–12 secs	+++
		A2B	1:128	12–15 secs	++
	Monoclonal	B	1:256	3–4 secs	++++
		A2B	1:128	5–6 secs	+++
Anti-AB	Polyclonal	A1	1:256	10–12 secs	+++
		B	1:256	10–12 secs	+++
		A2	1:64	15–16 secs	++/+++
	Monoclonal	A1	1:256	3–4 secs	++++
		B	1:256	3–4 secs	++++
		A2	1:64	5–6 secs	+++

TABLE 22.6: Quality control of Rh antisera reagents (anti-D)

Parameter	Quality requirement	Frequency
Appearance	No turbidity, precipitate, particles or gel formation by visual inspection	Daily and with new lot/batch
Specificity	Positive reaction with known Rh positive red blood cell antigens (RR) and no reaction with negative controls (rr)	Daily and with new lot/batch
Avidity	Macroscopic agglutination with 40% red cell suspension in homologous serum/normal saline using slide test	Daily and with new lot/batch
Intensity	No immune haemolysis, rouleaux formation or prozone	With new lot/batch
Potency	Undiluted serum should gives +++ reactions in titre of 1:32 or 1:64	With new lot/batch

TABLE 22.7: Acceptable titres and avidity and intensity of Rh antisera reagents (anti-D)

Type of reagent	Type of red cells	Titre immediate spin	Titre after 30–45 min incubation	Avidity	Intensity
IgM monoclonal		1:64 to 1:128	1:128 to 1:256	5–10 secs	+++
Blend IgM and IgG monoclonal		1:32 to 1:64			
Blend IgM monoclonal and IgG polyclonal	Pooled O O cells/ R1R1 cells	Same as above	1:128 to 1:256	10–20	+++
Polyclonal Anti-D			1:32 to 1:64 in alb, enz or AHG test	60 secs	+++

In problematic ABO/Rh(D) typing

- Check with anti-A, anti-B and anti-Rh(D) reagents of two different companies/batches.
- Rh-positive and Rh-negative controls to be tested.
- Always use washed RBCs.
- Do forward/reverse grouping.
- Any doubt, repeat with fresh sample.

- Check for auto-agglutination.
- Coombs' test, PS study to be done. Detailed clinical history has to be taken.
- Du testing undertaken.

Enzyme Reagents

Enzymes like papain, ficin, trypsin or bromelin should be used for incomplete antibodies.

The reagents should give specific results with positive and negative controls. Working reagent has to be prepared according to standard method.

Enzymes aliquoted and stored in frozen state. Only required quantity for the day has to be thawed. Unused enzyme at the end of the day has to be discarded.

Personnel, Training and Development

The number of personnel working in blood bank should be as per guidelines. Qualification of personnel should be as mentioned in the guidelines for:
- Blood bank medical officer, nurse
- Technical supervisor and
- Technician

The personnel should be competent enough and should have undergone training in:
1. Specific to their work
2. Quality control procedures
3. SOPs
4. Competency evaluation
5. Personnel health
6. Safety measures

Standard Operating Procedures (SOPs)[39]

SOP is a document which contains detailed written procedures and instructions describing the stepwise procedure of performing the tests and procedures in the laboratory.

SOP ensures uniformity, consistency and control over the processes carried out.

The procedure described should be performed by all the staff in the same way without any deviation. This is to ensure high quality of standards.

SOP should be available on the working table (laboratory bench work manual).

SOPs are controlled documents and necessary changes can be brought only with permission of the head of the laboratory or laboratory quality manager.

Note: Also refer to Blood Bank Organization and its Management.

Donor Recruitment

Quality blood comes from the quality donors.

Hence donor recruitment should be viewed seriously and care for the following to be taken.

1. Policy to get and retain voluntary blood donor pool
2. Donor selection—questionnaire and pre-donation counseling and consent
3. Interval between donations
4. Physical examination—general fitness
5. Donor notification of abnormal testing (TTI)
6. Post-donation counseling and referral
7. Donor reactions—manage properly

Donor criteria to be followed are:

Age: 18–65 years.

Blood pressure: 100–140 mm Hg of systolic pressure, 60–100 mm Hg of diastolic pressure.

Pulse: 60–100/minute.

Weight with calibrated scale: >45/>55 kg haemoglobin >12.5 g/dL.

Blood group—slide or matrix get card method: Re-checked again with another method.

Platelet count more than 1.5 lakhs/cumm.

For other criteria refer to the topic on 'blood donation'.

Phlebotomy

Hospital infection control team should be involved.

Aseptic precautions should be taken. Spirit and betadine applied—leave for 30 seconds. Spirit and betadine should be applied in a circular motion from inside out.

Care should be taken while handling the blood bag and needle.

Blood should freely flow into the blood bag. The blood bag should be below the level of donor arm. Raise the cuff pressure to 60–70 mm Hg. Remove the clamp. Reduce the pressure to 40–50 mm Hg once the flow establishes. There should be continuous squeezing of the fist. The technician should continuously mix of the blood with anticoagulant in the blood bag. The time taken for whole procedure is <10 minutes. The exact volume of blood drawn is 350 mL ±10% for whole blood and for component preparation it is 450 mL ±10% blood.

Note: Also refer to Donor Health Screening, Donor Suitability Evaluation, Phlebotomy, Post-Donation Care and ADR.

Blood Bag Selection[40]

- Single/double/triple/quadriple with integral filters can be used according to the need of component preparation.
- Use single bag when components are not separated, for autologous transfusion or for therapeutic phlebotomy.
- Check the bag visually for leakage/anticoagulant turbidity should be checked.
- Defective bags should be discarded.
- CPD/CPDA1/SAGM anticoagulant can be used.
- Anticoagulant: Blood ratio has to be 14 mL anticoagulant: 100 mL blood.
- Volume of blood collected is 350/450 ± 10%.
- Donor's weight more than 55 kg, 450 mL can be collected.
- Donor's weight 45–55 kg, 350 mL to be collected.
- Enter the following data on donor card and register:
  - Type of bag
  - Manufacturer's name
  - Batch No.
  - Expiry date

Blood Bag Labeling[41]

- Numeric identification number to be written.
- Expiry date to be mentioned.
- Donor number on bag to be written.
- ABO group and Rh type to be mentioned.
- Volume of blood collected to be mentioned.
- TTI result to be mentioned.

- Labeling of pilot tubes.
- Traceability of blood bag.
- Label should be clear and readable.
- Also colored label is put for different blood groups as given below.
  - a. 'A' blood group: Yellow color
  - b. 'B' blood group: Pink color
  - c. 'O' blood group: Light blue color
  - d. 'AB' blood group: White color

Blood and Blood Products Quality Requirements

- All preparation procedures should be done in a sterile environment.

TABLE 22.8: QC requirements of whole blood, red cells and platelets

Parameter	Quality requirement	Frequency of QC
QC Whole blood		
Volume	350/450 ± 10%	1% of all units
PCV (Hct)	45–55%	1% of all units
Sterility	By culture	1% of all units
Infectious diseases	ELISA/as per guidelines	All units
Red cell concentrate (prepared from 450 mL)		
Volume	225–350 mL	1% of all units
Hct	65–75%	Periodically, 1% of all units
Leucocyte poor red cells		
Post-filtration/apheresis procedure	Leucocytes less than 5×10^6	4 units a month
Platelets (RDPs)		
Volume	50–70 mL	All units
Platelets counts	$3.5/4.5 \times 10^{10}$	1% of all units/ 4 units per month whichever is more
pH	>6	
Residual leucocytes	$<5.5 \times 10^7 – 5 \times 10^8$	
Platelets (SDPs)		
Volume	>200 mL	All units
Platelets counts	$>3.5 \times 10^{11}$	1% of all units/ 4 units per month whichever is more
pH	>6	
Red cells	Traces to 0.5 mL	
Residual leucocytes	$<5 \times 10^6$	

- Blood bags should have closed system.
- The personnel should be trained.
- All the equipment used for the procedure should be calibrated and well maintained.
- SOPs should be followed.
- Records and registers should be maintained.
- Preparation of the blood components should be within <6 hours.

Fresh frozen plasma: Frozen within 6 hours of collection, using –80 deep freezers or blast freezes, stored at –18°C and date of expiry is one year.

TABLE 22.9: QC requirements of fresh frozen plasma

Parameter	Quality requirement	Frequency of QC
Volume	200–220 mL plasma	1% of all units/4 units per month, whichever is more
Factor VIII	0.7 units/mL	Same as above
Fibrinogen	200–400 mg	Same as above

TABLE 22.10: QC requirements of cryoprecipitate

Parameter	Quality requirement	Frequency of QC
Volume	10–20 mL	1% of all units/4 units per month, whichever is more
Factor VIII	80–120 units/mL	Same as above
Fibrinogen	150–250 mg	Same as above

QC of TTI screening
- Controls to be included in each run.
- If minimum number of recommended controls not included in a run, test is invalid in spite of having normal acceptable range of control values.
- Kits to be used before the expiry date.
- For incubation time and temperature, follow manufacturer's instructions.

Safety in Laboratory[41]

Persons working in the blood bank may be exposed for infectious agents arising from blood and blood products especially the blood borne infectious diseases. Also they can be at risk by the chemicals. The environment in the blood bank is also at risk of being contaminated with hazardous material used and waste generated in the laboratory. Hence, safety of both staff and environment is essential and the following measures need to be taken.

1. Documentation of laboratory safety policies and procedures.
2. All laboratory personnel should be aware of these policies.
3. All laboratory personnel should follow safe hygienic practices and wear glove and protective clothing during working hours.
4. List of hazardous material should be listed and properly disposed.
5. Biohazard symbol should be used on all containers having hazardous material.
6. There should be proper preservation and security of specimens.
7. Laboratory personnel should be thoroughly trained to manage spillage of infectious material.
8. Adequate fire extinguishers should be available and staff to be trained for managing fire.
9. Accidental events should be brought to the notice of designated authorities with description of events and analysed periodically to prevent and control such events.

Internal and External Quality Control

There are two types of laboratory quality control programmes:
- Internal quality control
- External quality control

Internal quality control: The technical staff in the own laboratory checks the performance by themselves and evaluate the reliability of the techniques.

Immediate decision can be taken to accept or reject the test results/products on daily basis.

This is required for daily monitoring of precision and accuracy.
- *Accuracy:* This is closeness of the measured value to true value.

- *Precision:* This reproducibility of test results, may or may not be close to the true value.

External quality control: The same may be evaluated by the external agency. It gives comparison of the performance with many blood banks.

It also gives long-term accuracy and performance of the analytical method.

Thus the external QC:
1. Establishes inter blood bank comparability
2. Ensures credibility of blood bank
3. Ensures high standards of practice
4. Encourages to use standard reagents and methodology
5. Encourages to improve
6. Helps to identify common errors

Internal Audit[42]

The quality assurance programmes must be monitored and one of the most effective ways of assessing this is through a regular internal audit of all activities. Internal audits also provide opportunities to identify areas that need improvement.

Documentation

Documentation is to ensure traceability of all blood transfusion service activities. These include:
1. Development of quality manual describing policies, standards and procedures.
2. Documentation of all activities including SOPs, forms, labels, etc.
3. Maintenance of records.
4. Documentation regarding issue, use, etc.

Convalescent Plasma and SARS-CoV-2 (COVID-19) Antibodies

Introduction

Immunity is the body's ability to recognize nonself-antigens and to mount a response to a pathogen by producing antibodies to prevent them from causing illness or damaging the body.

An immune system may contain innate and adaptive components. The innate system is essentially made up of barriers that aim to keep viruses, bacteria, parasites, and other foreign particles out of the body, while the adaptive system is composed of more advanced lymphatic cells that are programmed to recognise self-substances and foreign-substances (antigens such as infectious pathogens) and to react appropriately. The **adaptive immune system**, also referred to as the **acquired immunity**, is a subsystem of this immune system that is composed of specialized, systemic cells (B and T cells) and processes that eliminate foreign antigens and any toxic molecules they may produce.

There are two types of adaptive immunity: Active and passive.

- **Active immunity:** Antibodies that develop in a person's own immune system after the body is exposed to an antigen through a disease or when the person get an immunization (i.e. a flu shot). This type of immunity lasts for a long time.
- **Passive immunity:** Antibodies given to a person to prevent disease or to treat disease after the body is exposed to an antigen.

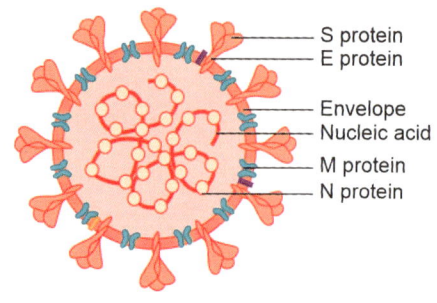

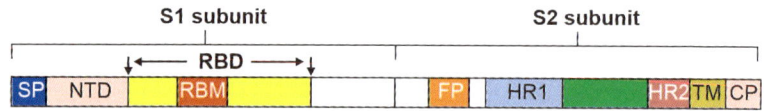

Fig. 23.1: Structure of coronavirus SARS-CoV-2

The novel coronavirus SARS-CoV-2, is an enveloped positive-sense single-stranded RNA viruses that with RNA size ranging from 26 to 32 kb are considered to possess the largest viral RNA genome. This large RNA covered with nucleocapsid (N) protein is held in a phospholipid bilayer and a complex of proteins including spike protein (S) hemagglutinin-esterase (HE) membrane (M) and envelope (E) which provide a crown-like shape for coronavirus. The S protein consists of two subunits: S1 and S2. The fragment located in the middle of the S1 subunit is the receptor-binding domain (RBD) in SARS-CoV, which binds to the host cell receptor angiotensin-converting enzyme 2 (ACE2).

SARS-CoV RBD contains a core and a receptor-binding motif (RBM); the RBM mediates contacts with ACE2. The surface of ACE2 contains two virus-binding hotspots that are essential for SARS-CoV binding.

Even though this particular virus is just about 13–14 months pathogen and the studies of the antibody response in infected patients are relatively new, yet the clinical values of antibody response are now being well understood. The antibody detection offers vital clinical information during the course of SARS-CoV-2 infection. The findings provide strong empirical support for the routine application of serological testing in the diagnosis and management of COVID-19 patients.

The present data demonstrated that typical antibody responses to acute viral infection are induced in COVID-19 patients. To be expected, the total antibody was first detected, followed by IgM and IgG. The seroconversion rate and the antibody levels increased rapidly during the first two weeks, the cumulative seropositive rate reached 50% on the 11–12 days and 100% on the 38–40 days.[43]

NEUTRALIZING AND NON-NEUTRALIZING ANTIBODIES

Serological tests are valuable particularly in epidemiologic studies and determining the immunity level of affected population including both diagnosed and asymptomatic individuals. Such studies also provide the primary platform for evaluation of the hypothesis like "herd immunity".[44]

Neutralizing antibodies (NAbs) are crucial in virus and bacterial clearance and have been considered essential in protecting against or preventing the spread of many infectious diseases. Passive immunity driven by CBP can provide these NAbs that restrain the infection. The RBD of the SARS-CoV-2 S protein is a major target for the antibody response. NAbs targeting SARS-CoV RBD generally prevent the attachment of the virus to the host cell by interfering with the binding of viral RBD to cellular ACE2 receptor.

Non-neutralizing antibodies (non-NAbs), also referred to as binding antibodies that bind to the pathogen but do not affect its capacity to replicate, might contribute to prophylaxis and/or recovery improvement. Moreover, other antibody-mediated pathways such as complement activation, antibody-dependent cellular cytotoxicity and/or phagocytosis may also promote the therapeutic effect of CBP.[3] In some studies it has been found that severe COVID-19 patients had a large amount of non-neutralizing antibodies, which may contribute to antibody-dependent enhancement of infection.

Further Understanding of SARS-CoV-2 Neutralizing Antibodies[46–49]

Extensive efforts have been made on understanding antibody recognition of the RBD at the molecular level. As of October

2020, structures of 22 different human antibodies in complex with the SARS-CoV-2 spike were available in the protein data bank (PDB). Three major epitopes on the RBD are recognized by the currently characterized SARS-CoV-2 neutralizing antibodies. Most of these antibodies are specific to SARS-CoV-2, but a few can also cross-react between SARS-CoV-2 and SARS-CoV. These antibodies can be clustered based on their interaction with three distinct RBD binding sites:

1. Receptor binding site;
2. CR3022 cryptic site; and
3. S309 pro-teoglycan site

Most of the antibodies that bind to these three sites show neutralizing activity with SARS-CoV-2. Moreover, antibodies that bind the CR3022 and S309 sites have a tendency to cross-react with SARS-CoV RBD, as compared to antibodies to the RBS, which are highly specific for SARS-CoV-2. Nevertheless, recent studies have indicated that the mutation do not change the antigenicity of the S protein and may even increase the susceptibility of the SARS-CoV-2 to antibody neutralization.

However, some minor natural variants with an occurrence frequency of <1%, including A475V, L452R, V483A, F490L, and H519P on the RBD, have been shown to alter antigenicity, as assessed by both monoclonal antibodies and convalescent sera. Escape mutations to monoclonal antibodies have also been identified by *in vitro* selection. These observations suggest that SARS-CoV-2 could undergo antigenic drift in the future if it becomes a seasonal virus.

Since the publication of the first structure of antibody in complex with SARS-CoV-2 RBD about an year ago, many other antibody structures that target the SARS-CoV-2 RBD have now been determined. This compendium of structures has provided important insights into the antigenicity and main sites of vulnerability on SARS-CoV-2. However, it remains to be seen whether all of the epitopes on the RBD have yet been identified and whether regions that are not currently known to be targeted by antibodies are truly non-immunogenic or elicit antibodies less frequently. Since most neutralizing antibodies to SARS-CoV-2 target the immunodominant RBD, structural studies have been focused so far on RBD-targeting antibodies.

It is remarkable how much structural information has already been amassed in such a relatively short time and a testament to prior investment in technologies, techniques and researchers by funding agencies and our institutions over the years for investigation of microbial pathogens.

Antibody Response to SARS-CoV-2 and Role of Neutralizing Antibodies in COVID Convalescent Plasma

In patients with SARS-CoV infection, B cell responses typically arise first against the nucleocapsid (N) protein. Within 4–8 days after symptom onset, antibody responses to S protein are found.[49,50] Neutralizing antibody responses, primarily to the S (RBD) protein, begin to develop by week 2, and most patients develop neutralizing antibodies by week 3.[51,52] Once such patients have recovered antibodies are likely to be effective against SARS-CoV-2. Plasma from donors who have recovered from COVID-19 contains neutralizing antibodies to SARS-CoV-2 virus that may help suppress the virus and modify the inflammatory response. Convalescent plasma has been applied with apparently good clinical results in COVID-19 and was also previously used successfully in the treatment of SARS.[53] While mechanistic correlates of protection have not yet been identified in humans, neutralization of the virus is presumed

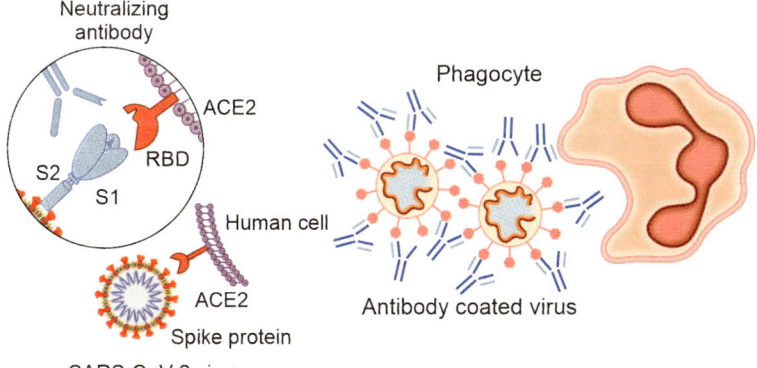

Fig. 23.2: Passively transferred neutralising antibodies react with spike protein of the virus. Antibody coated viruses form clusters gets recognised and phagocytosed

to be an important mechanism of action for antibodies, although the specific titre and specificity of the antibody repertoire required (for protection) remain debatable. In SARS-CoV-2, the primary target of neutralizing antibodies is the RBD, comprising 33 amino acids in the region (amino acids 460–492) amino acid region in the S protein, which can independently bind to the host target ACE2 receptor.[54]

Acquisition and Convalescent Plasma (CP) Use

The convalescent donors must undergo standard pre-donation assessment to ensure compliance with current regulations regarding plasma donation.[55] Currently, convalescent donors between 18 and 60 males and nulliparous females with weight >50 kg are considered as subjects without infectious symptomatology for COVID-19 after 14 days of recovery. The diagnosis of COVID- 19 infection can be either by COVID-19 RT-PCR or rapid antigen tests. IgG antibody against COVID-19 titre of 1:640 (ELISA) or 13 AU/mL (CLIA) or neutralizing antibodies 1:80 (PRNT/MNT) are recommended for donor selection. As CP production requires high quality standards, it must be free of any infection, so tests for human immunodeficiency virus (HIV), hepatitis B, hepatitis C, syphilis and malaria should be carried out.

Apheresis is the recommended procedure to obtain plasma. This procedure is based on a continuous centrifugation of blood from donor to allow selective collection plasma. The efficiency of this technique is around 400–500 mL from a single apheresis donation. This amount of plasma could be stored in units of 200 or 250 mL, and frozen within 24 hours of collection to be used in further transfusions.

There is no standard transfusion dose of CP. In different studies for coronaviruses the administration of CP ranges between 200 and 500 mL in single or double scheme dosages. Currently, the recommendation is to administrate 4–13 mL/kg per dose (usually 200 mL single dose) given slowly.

References

Journals Quoted in Text

1. Strobel E. Haemolytic transfusion reactions. Transfusion Medicine and Hemotherapy. 2008; 35:346–353.

2. Feroz A, et al, Blood Substitutes: Possibilities with nanotechnology. Indian J Hematology Blood Transfusion 2014: 30;155–162.

3. WHO Guidelines on Drawing Blood: Best Practices in Phlebotomy Geneva: World Health Organization; 2010.

4. India HIV estimation 2015 technical report, NACO and National Institute of Medical Statistics, Govt of India.

5. Guidelines for diagnosis and treatment of malaria, NVBDCP, New Delhi 2009, National Drug Policy on Malaria 2013, NVBDCP, New Delhi.

6. Snounou GS, Virixakosol S, Zhu X P, Jarra W, Pinheiro L, doRosario VE, Thaithong S and Brown KN. High sensitivity of detection human malaria parasites by the use of nested PCR. Mol Biochem Parasitol 1993; 61:315–320.

7. The Joint United Nations Program on HIV/AIDS (UNAIDS), Report on the global HIV/AIDS Epidemic 2003 and 2012, Geneva.

8. Weusten JJ, Vermeulen M, van Drimmelen H, Lelie N. Refinement of a viral transmission risk model for blood donations in seroconversion window phase screened by NAT in different pool sizes and repeat test algorithms. Transfusion. 2011; 51:203–15.

9. Red blood cell storage in SAGM and AS. Blood Transfusion 2012; 10 (suppl.):546–55.

10. Kasuya H, Onda H, Yoneyama T, Sasaki T, Hori T. Bedside monitoring of circulating blood volume after subarachnoid haemorrhage. Stroke. 2003; 34:956–60.

11. Cropp G J. Changes in blood and plasma volumes during growth. J Pediatr. 1971; 78:220–29.

12. Carson J L, et. al. Red blood cell transfusion: a clinical practice guidelines of the AABB. Ann intern Med 2012; 157:49–58.

13. Appropriate Use of Blood and Blood Products. The Kenya National Blood Transfusion Service, 2004.

14. Guidelines for the Appropriate Use of Blood and Blood Products. Second Edition, 2004 American College of Surgeons Adv Trauma Life Supp.

217

15. Simon Tl, et. al. Practice parameter for the use of red blood cell transfusions: developed by the red blood cell administration practice guideline development task force of the College of American Pathologists. Arch Pathol Lab Med 1998; 122:130–8.

16. Practice guidelines for perioperative blood transfusion and adjuvant therapies: an updated report by the American Society of Anesthesiologist's task force on perioperative blood transfusion and adjuvant therapies. Anesthesiology 2006; 105:198–208.

17. Ferraris V A, et.al. Perioperative blood transfusion and blood conservation in cardiac surgery: the Society of Thoracic Surgeons and the Society of Cardiovascular Anesthesiologists clinical practice guideline. Ann thorac surg 2007; 83:S27–S86.

18. Retter A et al. Guidelines on the management of anaemia and red cell transfusion in adult critically ill patients. British J of Haematology, 2013; 160:445–464.

19. Carson JL, et. al. Clinical Practice Guidelines from the AABB: Red Blood Transfusion thresholds and storage JAMA. 2016;316:2025–35.

20. Platelet Transfusion: A Clinical Practice Guideline from the AABB, Ann Intern Med. 2015; 162:205–13.

21. RCOG Guidelines in Obstetrics, RCOG Green top guidelines No. 47, 2008.

22. Paediatr Child Health 2014;19(4);213–17.

23. Jain R, Jose B, Coshic P, Agarwal R, Deorari AK, Blood and blood component therapy in neonates, AIIMS-NICU protocols 2008, Indian J of Pediatrics 2008; 75:489–495.

24. Canadian Blood Services. Clinical guide to transfusion Medicine, 2013.

25. Strauss RG. How I Transfuse Red Blood Cells and Platelets to Infants Transfusion 2008; 48:209–217.

26. Strauss RG. Platelet Transfusion in Neonates (Editorial) Expert Rev. Hematol 2010: 3:7–9.

27. Murray N A, Roberts IAG. Neonatal transfusion practice. Arch Dis Child FN 2004; 89:101–107.

28. Roseff SD, et al. Guidelines for assessing appropriateness of pediatric transfusion 2002; 42:1398–1413.

29. AABB press 2009.

30. Saricaoglu F, et. al., The effect of acute normovolemic hemodilution and acute hypovolemic hemodilution on coagulation and allogenic transfusion. Saudi Med J 2005; 26:792–798.

31. Terai A, et. al., Use of ANH in patients undergoing radical prostatectomy. Urology 2005; 65:1152–1156.

32. National Blood Policy 2007.

33. Mallik V. Laws relating to Drugs and Cosmetics, 22nd Edn. 2011 Eastern Book Company, Lucknow, India

34. NACO, Ministry of Health and Family Welfare, New Delhi 2007.

35. Wong KF. Virtual Blood Bank Journal of Pathology Informatics, 2011; 2:6.

36. Wong KF and Angela MY Kwan. Virtual Blood Banking: A 7 years' Experience Am J Clin Pathol 2005; 124:124–128.

37. Coustasse A, Meadows P, Hall RS , Hibner T, Deslich S. Utilizing Radiofrequency Identification Technology to Improve Safety and Management of Blood Bank Supply Chains. Telemed J E Health. 2015 Nov; 21(11):938–45.

38. Vox Sanguinis. Guidelines for the use of RFID technology in blood transfusion, journal compilation 2010, ISBT: 98 suppl 2:1–24.

39. Guidelines for Good Clinical Laboratory Practices, ICMR 2008.

40. WHO New Delhi.

41. WHO Bhutan.

42. VA. Armstrong Quality assurance in blood banking: the basis for safety Journal compilation, International Society of Blood Transfusion, ISBT Science Series 2009; 4:2.81–285.

43. Clin Infect Dis, 2020 Nov 19; 71(16):2027–2034. Antibody Responses to SARS-CoV-2 in Patients With Novel Coronavirus Disease 2019.

44. Human Antibodies, Vol 28, no. 4, pp. 287–297, 2020, COVID-19: Significance of antibodies.

45. Transfus Clin Biol, Plasma Therapy Against Infectious Pathogens, as of Yesterday, Today and Tomorrow.

46. Cell 2021 Jan 21;184(2):476–488.e11, COVID-19-neutralizing antibodies predict disease severity and survival.

47. Recognition of the SARS-CoV-2 receptor binding domain by neutralizing antibodies, Biochemical and Biophysical Research Communication.

48. Nature, volume 581, pages 221–224 (2020). Structural basis of receptor recognition by SARS-CoV-2.

49. Tan, YJ et al. Profiles of antibody responses against severe acute respiratory syndrome coronavirus recombinant proteins and their potential use as diagnostic markers. Clin. Diagn. Lab. Immunol. 11, 362–371 (2004).

50. Wu, HS et al. Early detection of antibodies against various structural proteins of the SARS-associated coronavirus in SARS patients. J. Biomed. Sci. 11, 117–126 (2004).

51. Nie, Y et al. Neutralizing antibodies in patients with severe acute respiratory syndrome-associated coronavirus infection. J. Infect. Dis. 190, 1119–1126 (2004).

52. Temperton, NJ et al. Longitudinally profiling neutralizing antibody response to SARS coronavirus with pseudotypes. Emerg. Infect. Dis. 11, 411–416 (2005).

53. Xinhua. China puts 245 COVID-19 patients on convalescent plasma therapy. Xinhuanet http://www.xinhuanet.com/english/2020-02/28/c_138828177. htm (2020).

54. Xiao, X, Chakraborti, S, Dimitrov, AS, Gramatikoff, K and Dimitrov, D.S. The SARS-CoV S glycoprotein: expression and functional characterization. Biochem. Biophys. Res. Commun. 312, 1159–1164 (2003).

55. https://www.icmr.gov.in/pdf/covid/techdoc/ICMR_ADVISORY_Convalescent_plasma_17112020_v1.pdf

Books Referred

1. Napier JAF. Handbook of Blood Transfusion Therapy, 2nd Edn, John Wiley and Sons, Chichester, New York, 1995.

2. Rossi EC, Simon TL, Moss GS. Principles of Transfusion Medicine, Williams and Wilkins, Baltimore, 1991.

3. Petz LZ, Swisher SN, Kleinman S, Spence RK. Clinical Practice of Transfusion Medicine, Churchill Livingstone, New York, 1996.

4. Ruddman SV. Textbook of Blood Banking and Transfusion Medicine, WB Saunders Company, Philadelphia, 1995 and 2005.

5. Hillyar CD, Silberstein LE, Ness PM, Anderson KC. Blood Banking and Transfusion Medicine: Basic Principles and Practice, 2003.

6. Hoffbrand V, Daniel C, Edward G, Tuddenham D. Postgraduate hematology, 5th Edn, Blackwell publishing, 2005.

7. Godkar PB, Godkar DP. Textbook of Medical Laboratory Technology. 2nd Edn, Bhalani Publishing House, Mumbai, India, 2004, 867–869.

8. Lewis SM, Bain BJ, Bates I (editors), Dacie and Lewis Practical hematology. 9th Edn. Churchill Livingstone, 2004.

9. Stephen H. Robinson, Paul R. Reich. Hematology pathophysiological basis of clinical practice, 3rd Edn, Little, Brown and Company, 1993.

10. The Clinical Use of Blood WHO Handbook Blood Transfusion Safety. Geneva 2003.

11. Petra Seeber and Aryeh Shander. Basics of Blood Management. 2nd Edn. 2013 Wiley-Blackwell, USA.

12. Pediatric Transfusion: A Physician's Handbook, 2002.

Index

A and B antigens 41, 42, 45
A2B blood group 56
ABO antigens in secretions 47
ABO blood group systems 38
ABO discrepancy 48, 162
ABO system 41
Accreditation 180
Acute normovolaemic
 haemodilution (ANH) 151
Acute TR—immunological 78
  acute haemolytic transfusion
   reactions (AHTRs) 83
  allergic reactions 81
  anaphylactic and anaphylactoid
   reactions 82
  febrile non-haemolytic trans-
   fusion reaction (FNHTR) 79
  transfusion related acute lung
   injury (TRALI) 86
Acute TR—non-immunological 78
  bacterial contamination 87
  metabolic derangements 90
  physical and chemical
   haemolysis 90
  transfusion-associated circulatory
   overload (TACO) 89
Additive red cells suspensions 117
Additive solutions 108
Adverse donor reactions 36
Adverse effects and management 4
Aims of blood donation 16
Alloimmunisation 13
Amount of blood donated 16
Antepartum haemorrhage 136
Anti-A1 antibodies 56
Anti-A1 lectin—*Dolichos biflorus* 55

Antibodies 42
Antigens on leukocytes
 and platelets 156
Antiglobulin reagents 63
Antiglobulin test 66
Artificial RBCs 155
Association of blood groups
 with diseases 46

Bacterial testing 192
Barcode scanning 188
Blood and blood product
 quality requirements 207
Blood as a drug 195
Blood bag labelling 206
Blood bag selection 206
Blood bank refrigerator 199
Blood donation/collection room 173
Blood group antigens 42, 45
Blood groups similar to Rh 69
Blood transfusion in
  anaemia 125
  paediatric patients 145
Bombay blood group 47, 56
BP apparatus 199
Building 172

Care to be taken before transfusing 1
Cell salvage 149
Clinically important subgroups 55
Common signs and
 symptoms of TR 79
Component separation room 117
Components 113
  cryo-poor plasma 177
  cryoprecipitate 112
  fresh blood 116

fresh frozen plasma 122
granulocyte concentrate 177
packed red cells 117
platelet concentrates 121
platelet rich plasma 115
Confidential unit exclusion 32
Continuous quality
  improvement 196
Coombs' test
  direct and indirect 68
  procedure 68
Counseling for reactive donors 18
Criteria for donor selection 21
Crossmatching 73
Cryoprecipitate 111

DAT/direct Coombs' test 68
Decastello and Sturli 38
Deferrals 23
Deglycerolized/frozen red
  blood cells 104, 119
Delayed TR—non-immunological
  iron overload 119, 93
  transfusion transmitted
  diseases (TTDs) 95
Delayed TR—immunological
  post-transfusion purpura 92
  transfusion-associated graft-
  versus-host disease
  (TA-GVHD) 91
Demographic information 22
Different blood group systems 40
Different methods of
  autologous BT 148
Directed donation 19
Discovery of D antigen 58
Documentation 210
Documentation and
  record maintenance 179
Donor area 173
Donor health history and
  donor safety 31

Donor health history and
  recipient safety 31
Donor motivation 182
Donor physical examination 32
Donor reactions and
  management 28
Donor record maintenance 187
Donor recruitment and
  donor criteria 205
Donor screening 22, 30
Duffy system 40, 50
Du—weaker variant of D 61

Ensuring safety during
  blood donations 186
Equipment 173
Equipment in blood
  donation room 173
Equipment in component
  separation room 177
Essential steps in donor
  motivation 183
Estimation of blood loss 136

False negative Coombs' test 71
False positive Coombs' test 71
FFP storage 122
Forward grouping 51
Fresh blood 116
Fresh frozen plasma 112
Frog leap technique 150

General guidelines 172
Genetics 43
Granulocyte preservation 111

H antigen 44
Haemoglobin-based oxygen
  carriers (HBOCs) 152
Hb estimation copper sulphate
  method 21
Hepatitis B virus infection 101
Hepatitis C virus infection 101

History of blood groups 38
HIV infection 99
HIV positive patients 100, 18
HLA antigens 156

IAT, indirect Coombs' test 66
Implications of
 leukocyte antigens 156
Implications of platelet antigens 156
Importance of ABO grouping 41
Importance of blood donation 15
Indian blood group 41
Indications of red cell transfusion 124
Informed consent 23
Instructions to the donor 28
Internal and external QC 209
Internal audit 210

Karl Landsteiner 38, 39
Karl Landsteiner, Alex Wiener,
 Philip Levine and RE Stetson 38
Kell system 49
Kidd (Jk) system 50

Laboratory testing of ABO 51
Laboratory tests 23
Lectins 44
Legislation 194, 195
Leucocyte-depleted (reduced)
 red cells 8, 80, 118, 119
Lewis system 50
Lipid membrane artificial cells 155
Lutheran (Lu) system 40, 49

Major crossmatch 73
Major crossmatch by
 matrix gel system 73
Malaria 95, 97
Massive haemorrhage 128
Matrix gel card method 52
Matrix gel system for Rh typing
McLeod syndrome 50
Medical examination room 173
Medical history 22

Medicolegal concerns
 and ethical aspects 178
Minor crossmatch 73
MNSs system 49
Monospecific antiglobulin 64

NABH 194
NACO 195
National Blood Policy 171, 194
Neonatal transfusion 138

Organisational management 171

P system 49
Packed red blood cells 117
Para-Bombay phenotypes 47
Perflurocarbon emulsions 154
Peripartum/postpartum
 haemorrhage 136
Personnel, training
 and development 204
Phlebotomy 33
Physical examination 23
Plastic bags 109
Platelet preparations 121
Platelet preservation 121
Poly-specific antiglobulin 65
Post-donation care 35
Pre-operative autologous
 donation (PAD) 149
Preservative solutions 105
Pre-storage filtration for
 leucocyte reduction 8, 80, 119

QC of TTI screening 208
Quality assurance 193
Quality control 193
 of reagents 200

RDP and rise of platelets 3
Reagent storage and
 stability of AHG 65
Reagents and materials 199
Reasons for separation of
 blood components 113

Recent advances in
  platelet transfusion 192
Recombinant haemoglobin 155
Recovered plasma 111
Red cell freezing 110
Red cell transfusion
  in blood loss 126
Rejuvenate solutions 109
Rejuvenated red cells 120
Retaining donors 185
Reverse grouping 53
RFID 190
Rh factor 58
Rh locus 59
Rh system 49
Role of nanotechnology 155

Safe use of blood 1
Safety in laboratory 208
Sample collection and
  storage of AHG 65
Setting of blood bank 172
Significance of weak D
  in blood transfusion 41
Slide method of blood grouping 51
Smart blood bank
  management system 190
Spin-cool-filter method 119
Staffing pattern 175
Standard floor space requirement 173
Standard operating
  procedures (SOPs) 178
Standard thermometer 199
Standardization of AHG 64

Subgroup of ABO system 55
Syphilis 95, 103

Testing for Rh antigen 59
The blood vending machine 190, 191
Therapeutic plasma
  exchange (TPE) 134
TR and management 78
Transfusion in obstetrics 135
Transfusion of cryoprecipitate 134
Transfusion of FFP 133
Transfusion of platelets 130
Transporting blood and
  blood components 111
Tube technique of
  blood grouping 52
Types of donors 18

Ulex europaeus 44
Unexpected antibody reactions 169
Unexpected antigen reactions 169
Unit of blood and Hb rise 3
Universal donors and recipients 46
Unused donor units 190

Virtual blood bank 188

Washing of red cells 118
Weak or partial D 60
Weak variants of Rh 58
Weakly reacting or
  missing antibodies 163
Whole blood 116
World Blood Donor's Day 29